NEW DEVELOPMENTS IN MEDICAL RESEARCH

BLOOD DONATIONS

ATTITUDES, SAFETY AND FUTURE DIRECTIONS

New Developments in Medical Research

Additional books in this series can be found on Nova's website under the Series tab.

Additional e-books in this series can be found on Nova's website under the eBooks tab.

NEW DEVELOPMENTS IN MEDICAL RESEARCH

BLOOD DONATIONS

ATTITUDES, SAFETY AND FUTURE DIRECTIONS

ANTOINETTE LUNA
EDITOR

NOVA BIOMEDICAL
New York

Library of Congress Cataloging-in-Publication Data

Library of Congress Control Number: 2016941678
ISBN: 978-1-63485-457-3

Published by Nova Science Publishers, Inc. † New York

CONTENTS

Preface		**vii**
Chapter 1	Ethics and Blood Donation: A Brief Overview *Jean-Daniel Tissot and Olivier Garraud*	**1**
Chapter 2	Epidemiological Aspects of Hepatitis C Virus Infection among Seekers of Serological Tests in Blood Bank in Pará, Brazilian Amazon *Tiago P. O. Andrade, Adriana S. C. Pimenta, Priscila R. Rezende, Rubenilson C. Valois, José A. B. Crescente, Márcia F. M. Rojas, Márcia C. M. Chagas, Luciana M. C. Maradei-Pereira, José Alexandre R. Lemos and Aldemir B. Oliveira-Filho*	**9**
Chapter 3	Statistical Control of the Production of Blood Components Using Variables and Attributes Charts, and Capability Indexes *Paulo Pereira*	**27**
Chapter 4	Use of Modern Test Theoretical Instruments (Item Response Theory: IRT) at First Time in Objective Measurement of Nurses' Transfusion-Related Knowledge – A Hungarian Survey *Veronika Rajki and Mária Csóka*	**73**

Chapter 5 A Quantitative/Qualitative Approach to Better Understand the Donation Motivations of Apheresis Donors in Quebec, Canada **101**
Johanne Charbonneau, Marie-Soleil Cloutier and Balia Fainstein

Index **147**

PREFACE

This book discusses the global attitudes regarding blood donations, its safety and future directions. Chapter One provides a brief overview of the ethics of blood donations. Chapter Two focuses on the epidemiological aspects of the hepatitis C virus infection among seekers of serological tests in blood banks in Pará, Brazilian Amazon. Chapter Three discusses statistical control of the production of blood components using variables and attributes charts, and capacity indexes. Chapter Four demonstrates the use of cluster analysis and item response theory for the assessment of transfusion-related knowledge of nurses. Chapter Five reviews a quantitative/qualitative approach to better understand motivations of apheresis donors in Quebec, Canada.

Chapter 1 – Quality, safety, risks and risk management are currently the leading words in transfusion medicine, and several approaches are necessary to correctly evaluate the fundamental basis of blood transfusion. Ethics is probably the most focused approach with which to examine the inconsistencies and conflicts of interest of the various stakeholders involved in the transfusion medicine field.

Chapter 2 – Viral transmission by blood transfusion basically requires that the donor has an agent circulating in their blood, serological or molecular screening tests not be able to detect it and that the host is likely. Minimize the possibility of viral transmission by blood transfusion requires actions that can ensure the safety of the blood that will be transfused. These actions involve the capture of candidates for blood donation, check clinical and epidemiological, and molecular and serological screening of blood donors. In Pará, the epidemiological situation of HCV infection is not well known. Some studies have detected high prevalence of HCV infections in blood donors and patients with multiple blood transfusions, especially caused by genotype 1. Knowing the risk of transmission of HCV genotype 1 and the need to increase the quality and safety of blood units collected in Pará, the authors determined the prevalence, genotypic distribution and associated factors for HCV infection in seekers of serological tests attended at blood bank of the state of Pará, Brazilian Amazon. This cross-sectional study of non-probabilistic convenience sample was composed of individuals who donated blood for the purpose of obtaining the results of serological tests (test-seeking blood donors – TSBD), from January 2006 to December 2011, in blood bank of the state of Pará (HEMOPA), the largest blood bank of Brazilian Amazon. All samples of TSBD were tested for HCV antibodies and HCV RNA. All positive samples were genotyped using nucleotide sequencing and phylogenetic analysis of 5'UTR. All TSBD completed a questionnaire about possible risk factors for HCV infection. The data were evaluated using simple and multiple logistic regressions. In 473,632 blood donors attended by HEMOPA from 2006 to 2011, 496 TSBD were identified. Most TSBD were male (71.4%) with more than 12 years of education (high school and/or more completed). The mean age was 29.3 years (19-58 years, ±9.4 years). One hundred and five TSBD were positive for anti-HCV antibodies by EIA. Twenty-six TSBD had discordant results between EIA and real-time PCR. The HCV RNA was detected in 79 TSBD by real-time PCR. There was a predominance of infections caused by subtype 1a (64.6%) and 1b (31.6%). Subtype 3a (3.8%) was also detected. Statistical modeling was performed using the results of EIA and PCR. In both models, the factors associated with HCV infection were: education ≥12 years of study, monthly income ≤R$1,000/US$250, tattoos, and use of illicit drugs (intravenous/sniffing). This study identified important epidemiological information of HCV infection in seekers of serological tests in blood bank in Pará. This information highlight the potential risk that these blood donors represents for transfusion safety, especially to transfusional transmission of HCV.

Chapter 3 – The control of blood components quality is a requirement generalized in Europe by the European Commission Directives and in the Unites States by the American Association of Blood Banks standards. The use of a statistical process control methodology is recommended in the related literature, such as the European Directorate for the Quality of Medicines & HealthCare guideline to blood establishments. However, a correct statistical process control methodology is not systematically applied. Commonly, the control methodology is uniquely oriented to verify the compliance with specifications per individual component and to measure the number of defective components usually monthly. This is a serious limitation to detect unnatural patterns and to assure that the production has a non-significance chance to manufacture nonconforming components. This Chapter is based in a long-period practice in blood establishment, proposing answers to some questions related to the discussion and implementation of a statistical process control procedure. The reader could easily test the approaches using the provided data.

Chapter 4 – The role of nurses in transfusion therapy continues to increase. A set of reliable measurement tools is required to assess various components of the professional knowledge including factual knowledge, skills and competence as outcomes of nursing education and training. Traditional questionnaires and test methods do not allow the measurement of these characteristics properly, as these tools typically provide overall scores without relevant insight into areas in which nurses perform well, and those where their knowledge and/or skills should be improved substantially. Our nationwide survey took place between November 19, 2014 and February 20, 2015. Data were collected using paper-form and web-based anonymous, self-administered questionnaire. 657 nurses who were involved in transfusion therapy with changing regularity in adult in-patient wards took part in the survey. Data were processed using descriptive statistical methods. The knowledge and skills of 657 participants were assessed using a validated instrument consisting of a set of questions covering every aspects of transfusion therapy. The answers to these items were evaluated on a binary scale. Recorded answers of the participants were analyzed using hierarchical cluster analysis and item response theory tools such as the one-parametric Rasch model suitable for dichotomous data. Data analysis was performed with the SPSS program and the ltm module of the R statistical program. It was found that the transfusion therapy related knowledge of nurses was very incomplete (50.72%), and only about half of the nurses (52.3%) systematized the nursing functions correctly. The vast majority of the institutions had their own protocol, but responsible nurses assigned for transfusion care were present only in 23.9% of the wards. The paper presents the distribution of correct and incorrect answers to various questions about transfusion therapy along with the corresponding logit values and odds ratios, respectively. The characteristic curves of each item were determined on the basis of the number of correct answers that have been recorded. These curves highlight which questions were answered easily and which items were found harder to answer by the nurses who participated in the survey. In addition to the separate analysis of individual questions, a set of response patterns is also presented which shows how frequently the nurses responded correctly to different combinations (sub-sets) of questions. On the whole, nurses exhibited medium level performance in terms of knowledge and skills required for efficient and safe transfusion practice. The authors conclude that the identified problems can be resolved by improving professional responsibility of nurses, increasing supervision by nursing leaders and appropriate transfusiology training and regular retrainings. Objective and reliable measurement of the level of acquired knowledge is a key requirement in nursing education. This paper, which demonstrates the use of cluster analysis and item response theory for the assessment of transfusion-related knowledge of nurses, focuses on this issue for the first time in nursing research. The results of this survey have revealed substantial limitations and deficiencies both in knowledge and skills of nurses which need to be addressed by training in order to improve the efficiency and safety of transfusion therapy.

Chapter 5 – It is important to acquire a better understanding of the motivations of apheresis blood donors, especially in a voluntary and non-remunerated context. In 2014, the authors conducted a questionnaire-based survey in order to compare whole-blood donors' motivations for donating blood to those of plasma and platelet donors. To better interpret the responses provided in this study, the authors then conducted semi-structured qualitative interviews with 50 PPDs. For the first study, 795 whole-blood donors and 473 apheresis donors filled out a questionnaire in which they were asked to provide their motivations for donating blood. Descriptive statistics were carried out. An analysis of variance (ANOVA) was completed to determine which motivators strike out between the two groups. For the second study, 50 PPDs were invited to comment on the five answer choices retained in the questionnaire-based survey. A classification grid was created, based on the 22 items proposed to respondents as motivations for donating blood. 80% of all respondents selected "My blood can save lives" in their motivators' list. When comparing results, 12 motivators are shown to be statistically different between WBDs and PPDs. For example, 61% of PPD respondents chose "Helping other people is in my nature" as one of their five most important motivators. Almost half of them also selected "I think there is a strong need for blood products" (47%) and "It gives me a sense of pride" (45%) as major motivators. The results of the interview survey suggest, for example, that the most frequently selected motivator ("My blood can save lives") has been related to many situations. Among them: 1) Being directly informed by the Blood collection agency's staff of the potential use of blood transfusions, 2) Knowing someone who has received blood transfusions, 3) Having a rare and sought-after blood type, or, 4) Having received this information from a family member who is also a blood donor. While being motivated to donate blood because "My blood can save lives" is usually interpreted as a prosocial motivation (altruism), the underlying situations rather evoke: a marketing communication strategy (1), indirect reciprocity (2), an expectation of recognition (3), or a social norm (descriptive norm) (4). A detailed analysis revealed that blood donor motivations are more complex than existing studies demonstrate. Our study is the first to combine a quantitative and qualitative approach, thereby providing a much more detailed look at PPDs' motivations for donating blood.

In: Blood Donations
Editor: Antoinette Luna

ISBN: 978-1-63485-457-3

Chapter 1

ETHICS AND BLOOD DONATION*: A BRIEF OVERVIEW

Jean-Daniel Tissot[1] and Olivier Garraud[2]
[1]Interregional Blood Service SRC, Epalinges, and Faculté de Biologie et de Médecine, Université de Lausanne, Switzerland
[2]Institut National de Transfusion Sanguine, Paris and Université de Lyon/Saint-Etienne, France

ABSTRACT

Quality, safety, risks and risk management are currently the leading words in transfusion medicine, and several approaches are necessary to correctly evaluate the fundamental basis of blood transfusion. Ethics is probably the most focused approach with which to examine the inconsistencies and conflicts of interest of the various stakeholders involved in the transfusion medicine field.

* This paper has been adapted from Donation: Blood, by Tissot JD, Garraud O, Lefrère JJ, Osselaer JC, in Encycopedia of Global Bioethics, Springer Science DOI 10.1007/978-3-319-05544-2_148-1 and from Ethics and Transfusion medicine, by Tissot JD, Garraud O, Lefrère JJ, Osselaer JC, in New Cannibal Markets: Globalization and Commodification of the Human Body, J.-D. Rainhorn and S El Boudamoussi (editors): Les Editions de la Maison de l'Homme, Paris, 2015. The paper is dedicated to the memory of Jean-Jacques Lefrère.

Keywords: altruism, anonymity, blood, blood transfusion, donation, essential medicine, ethics, non-profit, not for profit, remuneration, safety, quality, risk, risk management, World Health Organization

INTRODUCTION

Many different representations are associated with blood, blood components, and blood transfusion (Garraud et al., 2013a), and several questions emerge as soon as transfusion medicine is evoked: the scandals of contaminated blood are still remembered, and have definitively changed our societal appreciation of global safety. Blood safety is based on five pillars: i) infection-related safety based on epidemiology and monitoring of infectious risk; ii) immunological safety based on individualized or personalized transfusion medicine; iii) safety in procurement, to ensure a robust blood component inventory; iv) patient-focused blood management that aims to evaluate the needs of each individual patient; and v) ethics (Garraud et al., 2015).

BLOOD DONATION

The idea of taking blood from one individual to infuse it into another was developed by the ancient Egyptians. The word 'transfusion' stems from the ancient Latin *transfundo*. Early on, its generally recognized meaning was extended to include two different notions: the corruption of a population by mixture with foreigners, with sexual and hybridization connotations, and the transfer of a debt (Tissot et al., 2013a).

Blood donations are generally intended for transfusion into another individual which normally occurs in a context of mutual anonymity (Tissot et al., 2015). A donor may also pre-deposit blood or blood products to cover his or her own prospective needs. A third possibility is so-called "directed donation," in which a donor gives blood to a particular recipient. An alternative to this not-for-profit policy is "compensated donation," in which a recipient receives blood under the condition that one or several of his or her relatives make(s) donation(s) to compensate for the blood component being issued. Laws in most Western countries prohibit this type of donation because it does not respect the voluntary and anonymous basis of donation and is often considered as an impingement to solidarity. However, if "rare" blood groups are needed, direct donation is organized.

ETHICAL OBLIGATIONS

The ethical obligation of both transfusion medicine physicians and clinical/medical laboratory scientists at blood transfusion facilities is to provide, in a timely fashion, to any patient in need of blood, blood components that are safe and best suited to his/her clinical situation, and to secure the forthcoming donations and/or further transfusion recipient needs (notably by limiting the risk of alloimmunization). Blood transfusion facilities must rely on donors, whose blood or blood components are collected in optimal conditions with the greatest respect for the donor, and with the commitment of making the best possible use of this gift.

Globalization of the health market, merchandizing of the human body, and social inequalities must be taken into consideration when discussing blood transfusion. In the industrialized world, most blood donors are unpaid volunteers (voluntary non-remunerated repeat donors; VNRDs) who donate blood for a community supply (Tissot et al., 2013b). Although many individuals donate as an act of charity, in countries that allow paid donation, some "donors" (who should *stricto sensu* be renamed "sellers") receive some financial compensation. There are also incentives other than money, such as paid time off from work. In developing or recently industrialized countries, where established supplies are limited, donors usually give blood when family or friends need a transfusion (directed donation/reposition donors), with or without compensation.

The WHO recognizes that achieving self-sufficiency "in the supply of safe blood components based on voluntary, non-remunerated blood donation, and the safety of that supply are important national goals to prevent blood shortages and meet the transfusion requirements of the patient population." This issue is an important ethical aspect of blood transfusion (Rossi et al., 2011; Group, 2012; Dhingra, 2013; Garraud et al., 2013b; Lacetera et al., 2013; Follea et al., 2014; Tissot et al., 2015). The International Society of Blood Transfusion (ISBT) has also updated the ethical rules for blood donation and blood transfusion. Thus, the main concerns of national health authorities regarding blood and blood components are to maintain an adequate blood and plasma supply for patients requiring transfusion, to ensure the appropriate use and guarantee the safety of blood products, and to prevent the transmission of infectious pathogens (Desborough et al., 2013; Herve et al., 2014). Epidemiological studies in the West have shown that blood obtained from VNRDs carries fewer infectious agents — as deduced from biological markers — than blood from paid donors. However, this finding does not necessarily have universal or eternal value (Ala et al., 2012).

Blood donation is developing in an era of a globalized movement of people, the ethical values of blood donations will certainly be challenged in the near future according to local practices and habits. Therefore, one should ask which value is to be prioritized between securing non-paid blood donations and providing blood to patients in sufficient quantity. Ethical judgment includes the balancing of two values (which, in a given context, may be conflicting) and the duty to evaluate the practical consequences of a choice. While respectable, the philosophical substrate intended by the concept of *solidarity* is linked to one's culture and is not necessarily universal (even the best intentions can in some cases lead to catastrophic events).

As already mentioned, whole blood can eventually be considered as a gift that is special in that it is a source of manufactured goods. Plasma collection by apheresis is more often the source of material designated for the industrial production of blood-derived drugs. Thus, in many parts of the world, individuals are paid to source plasma, which is then transformed into drugs. Globalization is highly present in the market of blood products, and business-related companies may be considered the new vampires of neo-colonialism. The situation may be illustrated as follows: the plasma of poor young individuals will be collected and treated to produce very expensive drugs that may eventually be useful for the elderly of the richest countries. This disaster scenario must be combated and condemned, as it violates all aspects of solidarity.

Obligations Towards Donors

Donors generously give time and blood; they have the "right" to do so in optimal conditions of safety and comfort, and to receive acknowledgement, and respectful explanation in case of deferral. They also deserve the best possible use of their donation and to receive all necessary information. According to a generally accepted rule in Western culture, the human body and its parts (including blood) cannot be the object of any kind of trade. However, the absence of remuneration does not imply that donors cannot have their travel expenses reimbursed. Indeed, not doing so might lead to social discrimination against the poorer blood donors. Offering donors tokens as signs of gratitude and friendship, and making soft drinks and snacks available to them, can hardly be seen as "payment" and is generally practiced. Nevertheless, certain individuals are entirely opposed, for personal "*ethical*" reasons, to any kind of reward, particularly special fancy entrées such as those created by well-known chefs. This extremist attitude is not easily understood by individuals having different cultural orientation. For instance, the Middle Eastern culture of gift exchange would probably not orient donors in Syria into thinking that they were receiving the gift in exchange for their altruism. On the other hand, a Syrian graduate student who donates blood in a western context but receives nothing in return may tend to interpret the interaction as inhospitality

The Nuffield Council on Bioethics report on "Human Bodies: Donation for Medicine and Research" has provided specific terminology and a rubric, termed an *intervention ladder*, regarding transactions made in connection with human bodily material, including blood and plasma. All relevant information is readily available on the website of the Nuffield Council on Bioethics. Several notions, such as "recompense" or "reward," have been redefined: a *recompense* is a payment to a person in recognition of losses they have incurred, material or otherwise, and may take the form of either reimbursement of direct financial expenses incurred in donating bodily material (such as train fares), or compensation for non-financial losses (such as inconvenience, discomfort, and time). A *reward* is a material advantage gained by a person as a result of donating bodily material, which goes beyond providing redress to the donor for the losses they incurred during the course of donation. If reward is calculated as a wage or equivalent, it becomes "*remuneration*."

The review of ethical principles and the proposed terminology regarding transactions involving human bodily materials led the Nuffield Council to envisage shifting attention away from the paid/unpaid donation dilemma toward making a distinction between altruistic and non-altruistic interventions. Altruistic interventions include information about the need for the donation of bodily material for the treatment of others or for medical research; recognition of, and gratitude for, altruistic donation through whatever methods are appropriate both to the form of donation and the donor concern intervention to remove barriers and disincentives to donation experienced by those disposed to donate, and interventions as an extra prompt or encouragement for those already disposed to donate for altruistic reasons. Non-altruistic interventions include those offering associated benefits-in-kind to encourage those who would not otherwise have contemplated donating to consider doing so, as well as financial incentives that leave the donor in a better financial position as a result of donating.

The Multidimensional Aspects of Ethics: Discrimination/Exclusion

Discrimination and exclusion represent the obscure face of blood donation. Deferral is aimed at securing the blood transfusion circuit and minimizing the risks for transfusion recipients. The paradoxes of the exclusion of men who have sex with men (MSM) are particularly difficult to address without reflecting on the many and particular ethical aspects of the question. Protecting public health is a legitimate public policy goal; however, permanently excluding gay and bisexual men, but not heterosexuals who have unprotected sex (and therefore pose an HIV risk), from donating is indeed questionable. Do people have the "right" – versus the "opportunity" or even the "chance" – to donate? However, *it is not the right of donation that should be discussed, but the right of patients to "benefit" from donated blood.*

Conclusion

Although health systems have developed ethics, economics have their own ethics as well. Blood products are very costly, and hospitals make every effort to limit the inappropriate use of such expensive blood components for clinical, ethical and financial purposes. *In fact, blood or blood components obtained from VNRD are not sold.* The price of these "goods" is in direct relation to all of the services and activities that are directly or indirectly required, from the promotion of blood donation to the transfusion of a blood component, and surveillance—a long chain of processes which are all controlled and traced.

References

Ala F, Allain JP, Bates I, Boukef K, Boulton F, Brandful J, et al. (2012). External financial aid to blood transfusion services in sub-Saharan Africa: a need for reflection. *PLoS medicine* 9: e1001309.

Desborough MJ, Murphy MF (2013). Legal and ethical issues in blood transfusion. *British J. Hosp. Med* 74: C2-4.

Dhingra N (2013). In defense of WHO's blood donation policy. *Science* 342: 691-692.

Follea G, Seifried E, de Wit J (2014). Renewed considerations on ethical values for blood and plasma donations and donors. *Blood Transfus.* 12 Suppl 1: s387-388.

Garraud O, Lefrere JJ (2013a). Blood and blood-associated symbols beyond medicine and transfusion: far more complex than first appears. *Blood Transfus.*: 1-8.

Garraud O, Lefrère JJ (2013b). Voluntary non-remunerated blood donation and reasons for donating: is there room for philosophy? *Blood Transfus.*: 1-2.

Garraud O, Tissot JD, Osselaer JC, Follea G, Vernant JP, Lefrere JJ (2015). Transfusion safety from the viewpoint of a musical quintet. *Blood Transfus.*: in press (doi: 10.2450/2015.0297-14.)

Group WHOE (2012). Expert Consensus Statement on achieving self-sufficiency in safe blood and blood products, based on voluntary non-remunerated blood donation (VNRBD). *Vox Sang* 103: 337-342.

Herve C, Tissot JD, Bouesseau MC, Pottier R, Monsellier M, Garraud O, et al. (2014). [Ethics and transfusion--seminar report]. *Transfus. Clin. Biol.* 21: 66-76.

Lacetera N, Macis M, Slonim R (2013). In defense of WHO's blood donation policy--response. *Science* 342: 692.

Rossi F, Perry R, de Wit J, Evers T, Follea G (2011). How expanding voluntary non-remunerated blood donations would benefit patients, donors and healthcare systems? *Vox Sang* 101: 176-177.

Tissot JD, Lion N (2013a). Myths: history, blood, sex and money. *Blood Transfus.* 11: 1-3.

Tissot JD, Danic B, Schneider T (2015). [Blood transfusion - safety of the inventory]. *Presse Med.* 44: 178-188.

Tissot JD, Garraud O, Danic B, Cabaud JJ, Lefrere JJ (2013b). [Ethics and blood transfusion]. *Transfus Clin. Biol.* 20: 423-439.

In: Blood Donations
Editor: Antoinette Luna
ISBN: 978-1-63485-457-3

Chapter 2

EPIDEMIOLOGICAL ASPECTS OF HEPATITIS C VIRUS INFECTION AMONG SEEKERS OF SEROLOGICAL TESTS IN BLOOD BANK IN PARÁ, BRAZILIAN AMAZON

Tiago P. O. Andrade[1], Adriana S. C. Pimenta[2], Priscila R. Rezende[2], Rubenilson C. Valois[2], José A. B. Crescente[3], Márcia F. M. Rojas[2], Márcia C. M. Chagas[2], Luciana M. C. Maradei-Pereira[2], José Alexandre R. Lemos[2,4] and Aldemir B. Oliveira-Filho[1,2,*]

[1]Institute for Coastal Studies, Federal University of Pará, Bragança PA, Brazil
[2]Center for Hemotherapy and Hematology of Pará, Belém PA, Brazil
[3]Nucleus of Tropical Medicine, Federal University of Pará, Belém PA, Brazil
[4]Institute for Biological Sciences, Federal University of Pará, Belém PA, Brazil

[*] Corresponding author: Aldemir B. Oliveira-Filho. Faculty of Natural Sciences, Institute for Coastal Studies, Campus of Bragança, Federal University of Pará (UFPA), Bragança PA, Brazil. Alameda Leandro Ribeiro, s/n. Aldeia. 68.600-000. Bragança, Pará, Brazil. Phone: + 55 91 3425 1209. E-mail: olivfilho@ufpa.br.

ABSTRACT

Viral transmission by blood transfusion basically requires that the donor has an agent circulating in their blood, serological or molecular screening tests not be able to detect it and that the host is likely. Minimize the possibility of viral transmission by blood transfusion requires actions that can ensure the safety of the blood that will be transfused. These actions involve the capture of candidates for blood donation, check clinical and epidemiological, and molecular and serological screening of blood donors. In Pará, the epidemiological situation of HCV infection is not well known. Some studies have detected high prevalence of HCV infections in blood donors and patients with multiple blood transfusions, especially caused by genotype 1. Knowing the risk of transmission of HCV genotype 1 and the need to increase the quality and safety of blood units collected in Pará, we determined the prevalence, genotypic distribution and associated factors for HCV infection in seekers of serological tests attended at blood bank of the state of Pará, Brazilian Amazon. This cross-sectional study of non-probabilistic convenience sample was composed of individuals who donated blood for the purpose of obtaining the results of serological tests (test-seeking blood donors – TSBD), from January 2006 to December 2011, in blood bank of the state of Pará (HEMOPA), the largest blood bank of Brazilian Amazon. All samples of TSBD were tested for HCV antibodies and HCV RNA. All positive samples were genotyped using nucleotide sequencing and phylogenetic analysis of 5'UTR. All TSBD completed a questionnaire about possible risk factors for HCV infection. The data were evaluated using simple and multiple logistic regressions. In 473,632 blood donors attended by HEMOPA from 2006 to 2011, 496 TSBD were identified. Most TSBD were male (71.4%) with more than 12 years of education (high school and/or more completed). The mean age was 29.3 years (19-58 years, ±9.4 years). One hundred and five TSBD were positive for anti-HCV antibodies by EIA. Twenty-six TSBD had discordant results between EIA and real-time PCR. The HCV RNA was detected in 79 TSBD by real-time PCR. There was a predominance of infections caused by subtype 1a (64.6%) and 1b (31.6%). Subtype 3a (3.8%) was also detected. Statistical modeling was performed using the results of EIA and PCR. In both models, the factors associated with HCV infection were: education ≥12 years of study, monthly income ≤R$1,000/US$250, tattoos, and use of illicit drugs (intravenous/sniffing). This study identified important epidemiological information of HCV infection in seekers of serological tests in blood bank in Pará. This information highlight the potential risk that these blood donors represents for transfusion safety, especially to transfusional transmission of HCV.

Keywords: HCV, blood donors, transfusion safety, Brazilian amazon

INTRODUCTION

Viral transmission by blood transfusion basically requires that the donor has an agent circulating in their blood, serological or molecular screening tests not be able to detect it and that the host is likely [8]. Minimize the possibility of viral transmission by blood transfusion requires actions that can ensure the safety of the blood that will be transfused. These actions involve the capture of candidates for blood donation, check clinical and epidemiological, and molecular and serological screening of blood donors [34]. These actions also become critical to detect and exclude people living in greater exposure to risk of infection. Several studies have shown that improving the profile of blood donors directly influences the quality and safety of units collected [4, 9, 33].

Blood donor habitual and spontaneous is the most desired and therefore one most likely to promote best transfusion safety [3, 13]. Among the mechanisms that may compromise the safety of blood transfusion process, the individual's unclear motivation in seeking the transfusion service in order to perform a blood donation may signal a potential risk [13]. In Brazil, several people seek the donation of blood to obtain results of serological tests for viral infections, especially HIV infection [12, 14]. The creation of centers for testing and counseling for infectious diseases decreased demand in seeking blood donation as a means of obtaining test results [3].

However, recently in the Brazilian Amazon has been reported young drug users infected with hepatitis C virus (HCV) performing blood donation in order to obtain the test results [25]. The prevalence of HCV infection in the Brazilian Amazon is the largest among Brazilian regions, with the highest prevalence observed in the states of Pará and Acre [17, 30]. HCV is primarily transmitted by via parenteral routes. Blood transfusions without previous HCV screening and reuse and sharing of gloves, syringes and other material that can become contaminated are the most commonly documented routes of HCV infection [1, 31]. Other routes of HCV infection, such as sexual and mother-to-child transmission have been reported, but less frequently [18, 35].

In Brazilian state of Pará, the epidemiological situation of HCV infection is worrying. Despite the reduction in the prevalence of HCV infection in blood donors, this Brazilian state was detected frequency of 93% of genotype 1, likely transmitted by sharing materials perforating and cutting in households and public [25, 26, 37]. Since, genotype 1 was found in all patients with multiple blood transfusions infected by HCV, indicating the occurrence of viral transmission from donor to recipient blood [32].

Moreover, a high prevalence of HCV infection was detected among users of illicit drugs in the state of Pará, mostly caused by genotype 1 and with evidence of viral transmission associated with tattooing, sharing paraphernalia of drug use and high time drug use [23, 24]. Knowing the risk of transmission of HCV genotype 1 and the need to increase the quality and safety of blood units collected in the Brazilian state of Pará, this study determined the prevalence, genotypic distribution and associated factors for HCV infection in seekers of serological tests attended at blood bank of the state of Pará, Brazilian Amazon.

METHODS

In state of Pará (Brazilian Amazon), the Centro de Hematologia e Hemoterapia do Pará (Center for Hemotherapy and Hematology of Pará - HEMOPA) is responsible for meeting demand transfusion total public and private hospital network. Furthermore, it is nationally recognized for offering quality products and services with high levels of user satisfaction. In the period from 2006 to 2011, HEMOPA attended approximately 470,000 blood donors through routine care and campaigns to attract blood donors in public and private institutions in the municipalities of Abaetetuba, Altamira, Ananindeua, Augusto Correa, Belém, Benevides, Bragança, Breves, Cametá, Capanema, Eldorado dos Carajás, Castanhal, Itaituba, Marabá, Marituba, Paragominas, Parauapebas, Redenção, Salinópolis, Santa Bárbara do Pará, Santarém, Santa Isabel do Pará, Santa Maria do Pará, Santo Antonio do Tauá, São Caetano de Odivelas, São Francisco do Pará, Soure, Tucuruí, Tomé-Açú, and Vigia de Nazaré (Figure 1).

In parallel, HEMOPA developed two research projects to determine risk factors for HCV infection among blood donors from 2006 to 2011. All candidates for blood donation were seropositive for HCV and approximately three times the number of blood donors (random selection) with HCV serology non-reactive responded epidemiological questionnaire containing several questions, among which the blood donation was being made only for obtaining the results of serological tests for infectious agents. Blood donors who responded that they were donating blood for only the serological test results were selected to participate in this study.

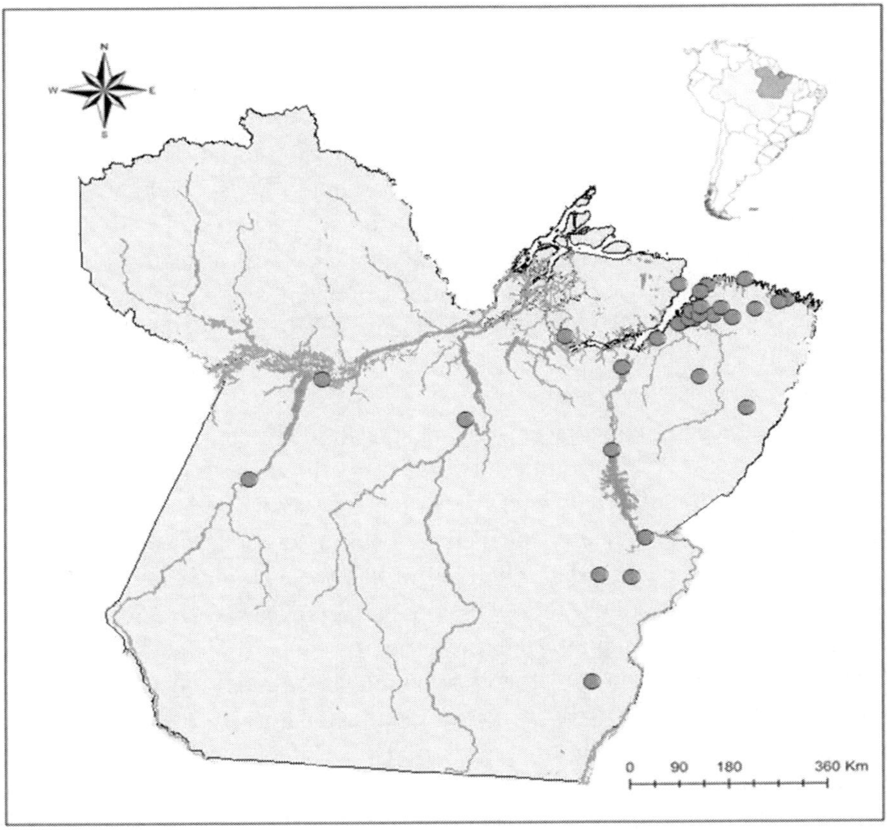

Figure 1. Geographical layout indicating the municipalities (•) where there has been captation of candidates to blood donation by HEMOPA in Pará, Brazilian Amazon.

Thus, this cross-sectional study of non-probabilistic convenience sample was composed of individuals who donated blood for obtaining serological tests related to infectious agents (test-seeking blood donors – TSBD) from January 2006 to December 2011. No blood donation provided by TSBD was transfused, independent of the results of serological tests.

All samples of TSBD were tested for Anti-HCV antibodies and HCV-RNA. Anti-HCV antibodies were tested by enzyme immunoassay (EIA - Murex anti-HCV 4.0, Murex Biotech, Kyalami, Gauteng, South Africa). HCV-RNA extraction was carried out from 140 μL of serum using QIAamp Viral RNA Kit (QIAGEN, Valencia, California, US), following the manufacturers instructions. Synthesis of the complementary DNA (cDNA) was made immediately after RNA extraction. Reverse transcriptase reaction was performed using High Capacity cDNA Reverse Transcription Kit (Applied Biosystems, Foster City, California, US), following the manufacturer's instructions. HCV RNA was detected by real-time PCR using 67 base pairs of the 5' UTR, as described elsewhere [27].

HCV-RNA-positive samples were selected for the amplification of the HCV 5' UTR using nested PCR [24]. The product of the second amplification was subjected to electrophoresis in a 2% agarose gel buffered with TBE and containing ethidium bromide, and amplicon DNA was visualized using an ultraviolet transilluminator. The amplified fragment was sequenced in both directions using the dideoxynucleotide chain terminator method in an ABI Prism 3130 system using a standard Big Dye Cycle Sequencing Kit, both supplied by Applied Biosystems.

All sequences obtained were edited and aligned using BioEdit software and the Clustal W algorithm, respectively. Phylogenetic analysis was performed by comparing sequences from the HCV 5'UTR determined in this study with HCV sequences deposited in GenBank, as described elsewhere [26]. Nucleotide sequence data obtained in the present study are available in the GenBank database under the accession numbers KX084715-KX084793.

All TSBD filled a questionnaire about possible risk factors for HCV infection. This collection tool for information had already been validated in other studies [25, 37]. Every possible risk factor for HCV infection were analyzed separately with the diagnosis of HCV infection by simple logistic regression to establish the p-value ($p < 0.05$), odds ratios and 95% CI. All of the potential epidemiological factors with p-values equal to or less than 0.2 during transversal tabulation were examined and controlled for in the procedures for the construction of the model of viral infection using multiple logistic regression with backward elimination in discrete steps (considering the p-value equal to or less than 0.05). The fit of final models were evaluated using the Hosmer-Lemeshow test. Two definitions of HCV infection cases were used: (i) anti-HCV positivity shown by EIA and (ii) HCV-RNA detection by real-time PCR. All statistical analysis was done using the software SPSS 18.0.

All participants signed consent term. All participants signed questionnaire with answers to population characterization and determination of factors associated with HCV infection. All participants received their results of laboratory tests. Participants with HCV infection were directed to reference centers for counseling and treatment of HCV infection in the state of Pará, Brazilian Amazon. This study was approved by the Ethics

Research Foundation Center for Hematology and Hematology Pará (01/ 2006-CEP/HEMOPA).

RESULTS

In 473,632 blood donors attended by HEMOPA from 2006 to 2011, 5,560 blood donors were positive for anti-HCV. In total, 23,265 blood donors (5,560 seropositive for HCV, and 17,705 with HCV serology nonreactive) responded epidemiological questionnaire about possible risk factors for HCV infection. Among these, 496 (2.1%) TSBD were identified. Most TSBD were male (71.4%), young adults (67.7%), married (59.0%), having monthly income of 1 to 3 minimum salaries (51.2%), and with more than 12 years of study – completed high school or more (61.0%). The mean age was 29.3 years (19-58 years, ±9.4 years). Table 1 shows characteristics of TSBD attended by HEMOPA in the state of Pará, Brazilian Amazon.

Moreover, one hundred and five (21.2%; 95% CI: 17.1-25.7) TSBD were positive for anti-HCV antibodies by EIA. The HCV-RNA prevalence was 15.9% (n = 79, 95% CI: 10.2-21.6). Twenty-six TSBD (5.2%; 26/496) had discordant results between EIA and real-time PCR. All TSBD were divided into groups, based on detection of anti-HCV antibodies (model 1) or HCV-RNA (model 2). In model 1, the case group consisted of 105 TSBD infected with HCV (presence of anti-HCV antibodies detected), and the control group consisted of 391 TSBD who were uninfected (presence of anti-HCV antibodies undetected). In model 2, the case group consisted of 79 TSBD infected with HCV (RNA-HCV detected), and the control group consisted of 417 TSBD who were uninfected (RNA-HCV undetected).

Using univariate analysis, several variables associated with HCV infection were identified: education ≥12 years of study, monthly income ≤R$1,000/ US$250, tattoos, and use of illicit drugs (Table 1). However, risk factors for HCV infection only began to be identified after multiple logistic regression analysis. Table 2 shows epidemiological characteristics associated with HCV infection in TSBD in the state of Pará, Brazilian Amazon (Table 2). The Hosmer-Lemeshow goodness-of-fit test showed a good fit for the final model 1 ($HL\chi^2 = 3.9$; $p = 0.6$) and model 2 ($HL\chi^2 = 3.2$, $p = 0.7$).

Table 1. Epidemiological profile of TSBD attended by HEMOPA, Pará, Brazilian Amazon

Variables	TSBD	%
Gender		
Female	142	28.6
Male	354	71.4
Marital status		
Married	293	59.0
Not married	203	41.0
Age (years)		
18-29	336	67.7
30-39	85	17.1
40-49	33	6.7
50-60	42	8.5
Education (years of study)		
Illiterate + less than 6	57	11.5
6-12	136	27.5
More than 12	303	61.0
Family income in 30 days*		
Less than minimum salary	34	6.9
1-3 minimum salaries	254	51.2
More than three minimum salaries	208	41.9

* Family income: average minimum salary from 2006 to 2011 = R$ 450.00 (about US $ 112.50).

Table 2. Univariate analysis of factors associated with HCV infection in TSBD in Pará, Brazilian Amazon

Characteristics	Overall sample	Anti-HCV+		HCV-RNA+	
	N (%)	*n* (%)	*OR* (CI 95%)	*n* (%)	*OR* (CI 95%)
Total	496	105 (21.2)		79 (15.9)	
Mean age (years)	29.3	27.5		27.3	
Age ≥35 years	107 (21.6)	21 (20.0)	0.9 (0.5-1.5)	17 (21.5)	0.8 (0.4-1,4)
Male	354 (71.4)	90 (85.7)	0.8 (0.4-1.6)	63 (79.7)	1.7 (0.9-3.1)
More than 12 years of study	303 (61.1)	88 (83.8)	4.2 (2.4-7.4)	69 (87.3)	5.4 (2.7-10.8)
Monthly income ≤R$1,000/US$250	232 (46.8)	69 (65.7)	2.7 (1.7-4.2)	52 (65.8)	2.5 (1.5-4.2)

Characteristics	Overall sample	Anti-HCV+		HCV-RNA+	
	N (%)	*n* (%)	*OR* (CI 95%)	*n* (%)	*OR* (CI 95%)
Supposed route of HCV infection					
Tattoos	83 (16.7)	50 (47.6)	9.9 (5.8-16.6)	32 (40.5)	4.9 (2.9-8.4)
Surgery	106 (21.4)	22 (21.0)	1.0 (0.6-1.6)	15 (19.0)	0.8 (0.5-1.5)
Recipient of blood transfusion	32 (6.3)	11 (10.5)	2.1 (0.9-4.4)	8 (10.1)	1.8 (0.8-4.3)
Invasive dental treatment	119 (24.0)	30 (28.6)	1.4 (0.8-2.2)	21 (26.6)	1.2 (0.7-2.0)
Uses needle/glass syringe at home	36 (7.3)	12 (11.4)	1.9 (0.9-4.0)	8 (10.1)	1.6 (0.7-3.6)
Shares razor blades in domestic environment/ barbershop/beauty salon	84 (16.9)	21 (20.0)	1.3 (0.8-2.3)	17 (21.5)	1.4 (0.8-2.6)
Does not use own nail clippers	185 (37.3)	43 (41.0)	1.2 (0.8-1.9)	31 (39.2)	1.1 (0.7-1.8)
Illicit drug use (intravenous/sniffing)	121 (24.4)	81 (77.1)	29.6 (16.9-51.9)	68 (86.1)	41.5 (21.1-75.4)
Unprotected sex	208 (41.9)	46 (43.8)	1.1 (0.7-1.7)	33 (41.8)	1.0 (0.6-1.6)
More than 10 sexual partners in the last 12 months	154 (31.0)	39 (37.1)	1.4 (0.9-2.2)	28 (35.4)	1.3 (0.8-2.1)

Table 3. Risk factors for HCV infection by multiple logistic regression

Risk factors	Model 1*		Model 2*	
	p-value	*aOR* (CI 95%)	*p-value*	*aOR* (CI 95%)
More than 12 years of study	<0.01	5.1 (1.9-8.6)	<0.01	5.3 (2.1-9.9)
Monthly income ≤R$1,000/US$250	0.01	3.1 (1.4-4.7)	0.02	2.2 (1.3-5.1)
Tattoos	<0.01	8.3 (3.4-17.2)	<0.01	5.1 (2.2-8.9)
Illicit drug use (intravenous/sniffing)	<0.01	34.1 (12.3-56.3)	<0.01	43.2 (18.5-78.1)

Note: EIA: Enzyme immunoassay; PCR: Polymerase chain reaction; ORa: Adjusted Odds Ratio.

* HCV infection based on EIA (model 1) and PCR (model 2) results.

Furthermore, a total of 79 nucleotide sequences of the 5' UTR of the HCV were isolated, of which 61 (77.2%) were identical, so only one representative was maintained for the alignment. Thus, the final alignment consisted of 40 nucleotide sequences (18 nucleotide sequences of GenBank, and 22 nucleotide sequences of this study). The Modelgenerator program identified the most adequate evolutionary model for the data matrix as the Tamura-Nei model adjusted by the parameters nucleotide frequencies, proportions of invariable sites, and gamma distribution rate. Base frequencies and transition/transversion rates for purines and pyrimidines were estimated by PhyML software during the phylogenetic analysis. The phylogenetic tree of the HCV affecting the TSBD revealed a marked prevalence of genotype 1 (96.2%, 76/79), followed by genotype 3 (3.8%, 3/79). While the bootstrap values were not significant (<95.0), the phylogenetic tree indicated a predominance of subtype 1a (64.6%, 51/79), followed by subtypes 1b (31.6%, 25/79), and 3a (3.8%, 3/79) (Figure 2).

Discussion

The prevalence of TSBD in the State of Pará (Brazilian Amazon) is less than in other studies. Using different definitions, the percentage of TSBD in the literature varies, being 2.0% in Zimbabwe [19], 2.8% in Norway [34], 5.9% in Hong Kong [16], 8.1% in Brazil [12], and 3·2% [7] in the US. Similar to other studies, most TSBD in Pará are men. However, several TSBD have many years of study and reduced monthly income. The good level of education and low monthly income may represent an indication that TSBD do not have enough income to carry out tests in private institutions, do not want to perform tests in the center of testing and counseling (public institution), and may be taking advantage of the idea of altruistic blood donation, often highlighted in funding campaigns of blood donors. An epidemiological study on factors associated with HCV infection among blood donors in Pará, initially, some participants omitted who had used illicit drugs [25]. This suggestion is possible to be occurring and should be evaluated in another study on knowledge, attitudes and motivations of candidates for blood donation in Pará. Among many characteristics observed in TSBD profile, some may be highlighted, such as: use of illicit drugs, unprotected sex, and multiple sexual partners. These characteristics are indicative of transfusion risk that TSBD may represent. The epidemiological features found in this group can contribute to transmission of many pathogens, such as HCV, HBV and HIV [6, 20, 25].

In summary, this study reinforces the idea that blood donors are not a homogenous group and motivation to come to blood centers may be associated with both individual and social group characteristics.

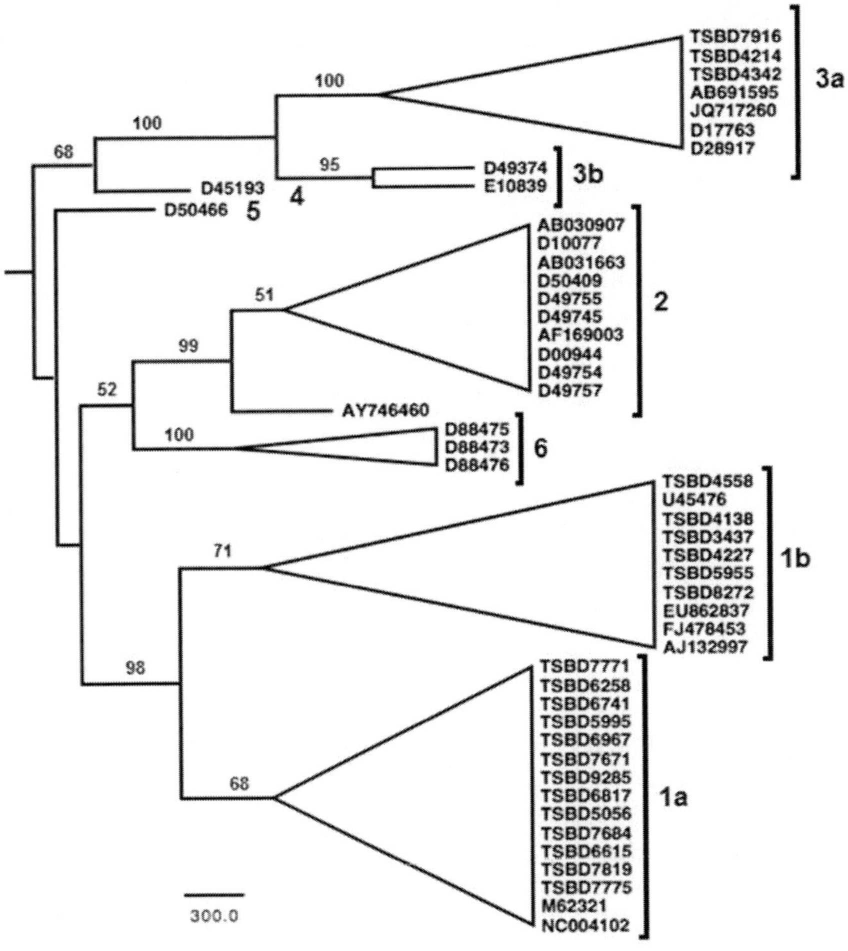

Figure 2. Maximum-likelihood phylogenetic tree derived from the alignment of 340 base pairs of the 5' UTR of the hepatitis C virus detected in TSBD attended by HEMOPA, Pará, Brazilian Amazon. The topological robustness of the tree was evaluated using a bootstrap analysis with 1,000 replicates (bootstrap values of less than 50 are not shown). The individuals selected for the present study are identified in the figure by TSBD + sample number.

Moreover, epidemiological studies on the prevalence of HCV infections have been conducted in certain populations in Pará. The prevalence of antibodies to anti-HCV among blood donors was 0.22%, and prevalence of HCV RNA was 0,13% [26]. In riverside communities, anti-HCV antibodies range from 2.2% to 8.8%, being detected the prevalence of HCV RNA of 5.5% among riparians [5, 21]. In patients with chronic kidney disease undergoing hemodialysis, the prevalence of antibodies to anti-HCV was 8.4%, and prevalence of HCV RNA was 4.6% [10]. The prevalence of HCV infection among illicit drugs users was higher, anti-HCV antibodies range from 32.3% to 35.3%, and RNA-HCV range from 28.0% to 31.3%. These variations in the prevalence of HCV infection reflect the evaluation of users of different drugs [23, 24].

In this study, the prevalence of anti-HCV antibodies (21.2%) and RNA-HCV (15.9%) among test seekers was high, indicating the vulnerability and the potential risk of transmission of HCV. In São Paulo (Southeastern Brazil), an epidemiological study with test seekers also identified high risk of viral infections, in particular microorganisms related to sexual transmission, such as HIV [12]. Despite the existence of testing and counseling centers, this study shows that it is still possible to detect tests seekers in blood bank in the state of Pará. Likely, measures to provide education and awareness of the candidates for blood donation on the benefits and risks of blood donation to receptors, associated with less bureaucracy to service at testing and counseling centers, can reduce the number of test seekers in blood bank. The improvement of the profile of candidates for blood donation impacts directly on quality and safety of collected units.

Moreover, this study determined four risk factors for HCV infection in TSBD. The educational level and family income are not properly risk factors for HCV infection. Likely, these features act as factors associated with other features. Many TSBD not want to perform tests to identify infectious agents in testing and counseling centers, they does not have enough family income to pay for such tests in private institutions, but they has the knowledge that blood banks conduct such tests with quality, and also will be very well received as altruistic blood donors. This hypothesis is supported by the identification of illicit drug use and tattooing as risk factors for HCV infection. These two risk factors for HCV infection are well documented in the literature, including epidemiological studies on vulnerable populations in Pará [24, 28]. The results of this study may show that users of illicit drugs, with reduced time of illicit drugs, little financial resources and good educational level are looking for the donation of blood to evaluate the acquisition of infectious agents. Epidemiological studies of illicit drug users in Pará are being conducted to evaluate this hypothesis.

Most hepatitis C infections in Brazil are caused by HCV genotypes 1, 2 and 3 [3, 17]. This study showed a predominance of genotype 1, followed by genotypes 3. In Pará and other states that constitute the Brazilian Amazon, genotype 1 has been found in higher frequency [3, 26, 29, 32]. Sawada et al. [32] indicated that changes in social behavior affect the epidemiological trends of infectious diseases to a significant extent, including the distribution of HCV genotypes. In spite of the reduced frequency of genotype 3 observed in this study, possibly, TSBD have contributed to the detection of genotype 3 among blood donors in Pará [26, 32].

This study has limitations. First, the definition of test seeker is difficult to validate. This study used one question to define test seeking. Thus, misclassification could have occurred due to the inability to know for certain which donors were actual test seekers. Another limitation may be due to employing an intentionally brief, self-administered questionnaire. There were not questions available to assess social capital. Thus, it was not possible to assess all dimensions of cognitive and structural social capital as described in the literature [15, 22]. A further limitation is that our findings are from State of Pará and may not be directly generalizable to other settings. Finally, modelling exercises have shown that an effect of test-seeking behaviour can offset gains in improvement of screening for viral infections [11]. However, we recognize that the association of test seeking with risk of viral infections needs to be confirmed prospectively.

CONCLUSION

This study identified relevant epidemiological information of HCV infection in TSBD. It determined a high prevalence of HCV infection compared to other epidemiological studies in Pará, as well as noted the predominance of genotype 1. In addition, it identified four factors associated with HCV infection: use of illicit drugs, tattooing, low family income and several years of study. These informations highlight the potential risk that TSBD represents for transfusion safety, especially to transfusional transmission of HCV.

Acknowledgments

Thanks to Andrea B. Neves (UFPA) and Danielly B. Oliveira (UFPA) for the collaboration in information collection and database assembly, and Adam R. Bessa (UFPA) for the elaboration of Figure 1. This study was supported by Ministry of Health, Brazil (PN-DST/AIDS-SVS/MS/BIRD/UNESCO-CSV 298).

Competing interests: The authors declare that they have no competing interests.

References

[1] Alter, M. J. (2011). HCV Routes of Transmission: What Goes Around Comes Around. *Semin Liver Dis.* 31, 340-346.

[2] Campiotto, S., Pinho, J. R., Carrilho, F. J., Da Silva, L. C., Souto, F. J., Spinelli, V., Pereira, L. M., Coelho, H. S., Silva, A. O., Fonseca, J. C., Rosa, H., Lacet, C. M., Bernardini, A. P. (2005). Geographic distribution of hepatitis C virus genotypes in Brazil. *Braz J Med Biol Res.* 38, 41-49.

[3] Carrazzone, C. F. V., Brito, A. M., Gomes, Y. M. (2004). The importance of pre-transfusional serological screening in blood transfusion recipients. *Rev Bras Hematol Hemoter.* 26, 93-98.

[4] Chandra, T., Kumar, A., Gupta, A. (2009). Prevalence of transfusion transmitted infections in blood donors: an Indian experience. *Transfusion.* 49, 2214-2220.

[5] De Almeida, M. K., Dos Santos, K. N., Fecury, A. A., De Oliveira, C. S., Freitas, A. S., Quaresma, J. A., Fuzii, H. T., Martins, L. C. (2012). Prevalence of viral hepatitis B and C in riverside communities of the Tucuruí Dam, Pará, Brazil. *J Med Virol.* 84, 1907-1912.

[6] De Almeida-Neto, C., Goncalez, T. T., Birch, R. J., De Carvalho, S. M., Capuani, L., Leão, S. C., Miranda, C., Rocha, P. C., Carneiro-Proietti, A. B., Johnson, B. R., Wright, D. J., Murphy, E. L., Custer, B., NHLBI Retrovirus Epidemiology Donor Study-II (REDS-II) International Component, Brazil (2013). Risk factors for human immunodeficiency virus infection among Brazilian blood donors: a multicentre case-control study using audio computer-assisted structured interviews. *Vox Sang.* 105, 91-99.

[7] Doll, L. S., Petersen, L. R., White, C. R., Ward, J. W. (1991). Human immunodeficiency virus type 1-infected blood donors: behavioral characteristics and reasons for donation. The HIV Blood Donor Study Group. *Transfusion.* 31, 704-709.

[8] Faber, J. C. (2004). Worldwide overview of existing haemovigilance systems. *Transfus Apher Sci.* 31, 99-110.

[9] Fasola, F. A., Kotila, T. R., Akinyemi, J. (2009). Trends in transfusion transmitted viral infections from 2001- 2006, Ibadan, Nigeria. *Virol J.* 13: 21.

[10] Freitas, M. J. R., Fecury, A. A., De Almeida, M. K., Freitas, A. S., De Souza Guimarães V., Da Silva, A. M., Da Costa, Y. F., Da Costa, R. A., Ferreira, P., Martins, L.C. (2013) Prevalence of hepatitis C virus infection and genotypes in patient with chronic kidney disease undergoing hemodialysis. *J Med Virol.* 85: 1741-1745.

[11] Glynn SA, Kleinman SH, Schreiber GB, Zuck T, Combs SM, Bethel J, Garratty G, Williams AE; Retrovirus Epidemiology Donor Study. (2002). Motivations to donate blood: demographic comparisons. *Transfusion.* 42, 216-225.

[12] Goncalez, T. T., Sabino, E. C., Murphy, E. L., Chen, S., Chamone, D. A., McFarland, W. (2006). Human immunodeficiency virus test-seeking motivation in blood donors, São Paulo, Brazil. *Vox Sang.* 90, 170-176.

[13] Goncalez, T. T., Sabino, E. C., Chen, S., Salles, N. A., Chamone, D. A., McFarland, W., Murphy, E. L. (2008). Knowledge, attitudes and motivations among blood donors in São Paulo, Brazil. *AIDS Behav.* 12: S39-S47.

[14] Goncalez, T., Sabino, E., Sales, N., Chen, Y. H., Chamone, D., Busch, M., Murphy, E., Custer, B., McFarland, W. (2010). Human immunodeficiency virus test-seeking blood donors in a large blood bank in São Paulo, Brazil. *Transfusion.* 50, 1806-1814.

[15] Krishna, A., Shrader, E. Social Capital Assessment Tool from Conference on Social Capital and Poverty Reduction. Washington, DC, The World Bank, 1999.

[16] Lau, J. T., Thomas, J., Lin, C. K. (2002). HIV-related behaviours among voluntary blood donors in Hong Kong. *AIDS Care.* 14, 481-492.

[17] Martins, T., Narciso-Schiavon, J. L., Schiavon, L. (2011). Epidemiology of hepatitis C virus infection. *Rev Assoc Med Bras.* 57, 107-112.

[18] Murakami, J., Nagata, I., Iitsuka, T., Okamoto, M., Kaji, S., Hoshika, T., Matsuda, R., Kanzaki, S., Shiraki, K., Suyama, A., Hino, S. (2012). Risk factors for mother-to-child transmission of hepatitis C virus: maternal high viral load and fetal exposure in the birth canal. *Hepatol Res.* 42, 648-657.

[19] Mvere, D., Shamu, R., Makoni, R., Lloyd, S., Nhau, E., McFarland W. (1996). Strong preference 'to donate' among HIV-positive blood donors in Zimbabwe. *Lancet.* 347, 902.

[20] Nascimento, M. C., Mayaud, P., Sabino, E. C., Torres, K. L., Franceschi, S. (2008). Prevalence of hepatitis B and C serological markers among first-time blood donors in Brazil: a multi-center serosurvey. *J Med Virol.* 80, 53-57.

[21] Oliveira, C. S., Silva, A. V., Dos Santos, K. N., Fecury, A. A., Almeida, M. K., Fernandes, A. P., Costa, C. A., Freitas, A. S., Corvelo, T. C., Martins, L. C. (2011). Hepatitis B and C virus infection among Brazilian Amazon riparians. *Rev Soc Bras Med Trop.* 44, 546-550.

[22] Oliveira, C. D., Goncalez, T., Wright, D., Rocha, P. C., Miranda, C., Capuani, L., Carneiro-Proietti, A. B., Proietti, F. A., De Almeida-Neto, C., Larsen, N. M., Sampaio, D., Custer, B., NHLBI Retrovirus Epidemiology Donor Study-II (REDS-II), International Component. (2013). Relationship between social capital and test seeking among blood donors in Brazil. *Vox Sang.* 104, 100-109.

[23] Oliveira-Filho, A. B., Sawada, L., Pinto, L. C., Locks, D., Bahia, S. L., Brasil-Costa, I., Lemos, J. A. (2013). HCV infection among cocaine users in the state of Pará, Brazilian Amazon. *Arch Virol.* 158, 1555-1560.

[24] Oliveira-Filho, A. B., Sawada, L., Pinto, L. C., Locks, D., Bahia, S. L., Castro, J. A., Hermes, R. B., Brasil-Costa, I., Amaral, C. E., Lemos, J. A. (2014). Epidemiological aspects of HCV infection in non-injecting drug users in the Brazilian state of Pará, eastern Amazon. *Virol J.* 11, 38.

[25] Oliveira-Filho, A. B., Pimenta, A. S., Rojas, M. F., Chagas, M. C., Crespo, D. M., Crescente, J. A., Lemos, J. A. (2010). Likely transmission of hepatitis C virus through sharing of cutting and perforating instruments in blood donors in the State of Pará, Northern Brazil. *Cad Saude Publica.* 26, 837-844.

[26] Oliveira-Filho, A. B., Pimenta, A. S., Rojas, M. F., Chagas, M. C., Crescente, J. A., Crespo, D. M., Lemos, J. A. (2010). Prevalence and genotyping of hepatitis C virus in blood donors in the state of Pará, Northern Brazil. *Mem Inst Oswaldo Cruz*. 105, 103-106.

[27] Oliveira-Filho, A. B., Oliveira, E. H., Castro, J. A., Silva, L. V., Vallinoto, A. C., Lemos, J. A. (2012). Epidemiological aspects of HCV infection in HIV-infected individuals in Piauí State, Northeast Brazil. *Arch Virol*. 157, 2411-2416.

[28] Pacheco, S. D., Silva-Oliveira, G. C., Maradei-Pereira, L. M., Crescente, J. Â., Lemos, J. A., Oliveira-Filho, A. B. (2014). Prevalence of HCV infection and associated factors among illicit drug users in Breves, State of Pará, northern Brazil. *Rev Soc Bras Med Trop*. 47, 367-370.

[29] Paraná, R., Paiva, T., Leite, M. R., Oliveira, F. N., Kali, N., Lobato, C., Dantas, T., Neto, J. T. (2007). Infection with hepatitis C virus among health care workers in the Brazilian Western Amazon region (Rio Branco, State of Acre). *Am J Trop Med Hyg*. 76, 165-169.

[30] Pereira, L. M., Martelli, C. M., Moreira, R. C., Merchan-Hamman, E., Stein, A. T., Cardoso, M. R., Figueiredo, G. M., Montarroyos, U. R., Braga, C., Turchi, M. D., Coral, G., Crespo, D., Lima, M. L., Alencar, L.C., Costa, M., Dos Santos, A. A., Ximenes, R. A. (2009). Prevalence and risk factors of Hepatitis C virus infection in Brazil, 2005 through 2009: a cross-sectional study. *BMC Infect Dis*. 13, 60.

[31] Prati, D. (2006). Transmission of hepatitis C virus by blood transfusions and other medical procedures: a global review. *J Hepatol*. 45, 607-616.

[32] Sawada, L., Pinheiro, A. C., Locks, D., Pimenta, A. S., Rezende, P. R., Crespo, D. M., Crescente, J. Â., Lemos, J. A., Oliveira-Filho, A. B. (2011). Distribution of hepatitis C virus genotypes among different exposure categories in the State of Pará, Brazilian Amazon. *Rev Soc Bras Med Trop*. 44, 8-12.

[33] Sojka, B. N., Sojka, P. (2008). The blood donation experience: self-reported motives and obstacles for donating blood. *Vox Sang*. 94: 56-63.

[34] Stigum, H., Bosnes, V., Magnus, P., Orjasaeter, H. (2001). Risk behaviour among blood donors who give blood in order to be tested for the human immunodeficiency virus. *Vox Sang*. 80, 24-27.

[35] Terrault, N. A., Dodge, J. L., Murphy, E. L., Tavis, J. E., Kiss, A., Levin, T. R., Gish, R. G., Busch, M. P., Reingold, A. L., Alter, M. J. (2013). Sexual transmission of hepatitis C virus among monogamous heterosexual couples: the HCV partners study. *Hepatology.* 57, 881-889.

[36] Tiwari, B. R., Ghimmire, P., Karki, S., Raj Kumar M. (2008). Seroprevalence of human immunodeficiency virus in Nepalese blood donors: A study from three regional blood transfusion services. *Asian J Transfus Sci.* 2, 66-68.

[37] Valois, R. C., Maradei-Pereira, L. M., Crescente, J. Â., Oliveira-Filho, A. B., Lemos, J. A. (2014). HCV infection through perforating and cutting material among candidates for blood donation in Belém, Brazilian Amazon. *Rev Inst Med Trop Sao Paulo.* 56, 511-515.

In: Blood Donations
Editor: Antoinette Luna
ISBN: 978-1-63485-457-3

Chapter 3

STATISTICAL CONTROL OF THE PRODUCTION OF BLOOD COMPONENTS USING VARIABLES AND ATTRIBUTES CHARTS, AND CAPABILITY INDEXES

Paulo Pereira*
Portuguese Institute of Blood and Transplantation, Lisbon, Portugal

ABSTRACT

The control of blood components quality is a requirement generalized in Europe by the European Commission Directives and in the Unites States by the American Association of Blood Banks standards. The use of a statistical process control methodology is recommended in the related literature, such as the European Directorate for the Quality of Medicines & HealthCare guideline to blood establishments. However, a correct statistical process control methodology is not systematically applied. Commonly, the control methodology is uniquely oriented to verify the compliance with specifications per individual component and to measure the number of defective components usually monthly. This is a serious limitation to detect unnatural patterns and to assure that the production has a non-significance chance to manufacture nonconforming components. This Chapter is based in a long-period practice in blood establishment, proposing answers to some questions related to the

* Corresponding Author address; Email: paulo.pereira@ipst.min-saude.pt.

discussion and implementation of a statistical process control procedure. The reader could easily test the approaches using the provided data.

Keywords: attributes, compatibility indexes, rational subgroup, sampling, sigma level, SPC, specifications, variables

1. Introduction

The control of the production of blood components is required in Europe by the Directive 2002/98/EC [1] and in the US by the standards for blood banks and transfusion services [2]. The European Directorate for the Quality of Medicines & HealthCare (EDQM) of the Council of Europe hosts the European Committee (Partial Agreement) on Blood Transfusion (CD-P-TS). EDQM publishes the "Guide to the preparation, use and quality assurance of blood components" [3], which includes in Appendix 4 a statistical process control (SPC) methodology. The Appendix is related to the implementation of SPC, schemes for statistical sampling (rational subgroup), regularity of control samplings, and a set of cases considering the use of charts, method of scan statistics, and a statistical process control for dichotomous results. However, the statistical monitoring of the blood components production is not currently a standardized practice.

Blood establishment policies should include quality control policies to assure blood components can provide to the receiver the therapeutic dose and to minimize the cost of poor quality. The management review should consider the control and the improvement of the blood components production. This monitoring and improvement should not be uniquely focused on the expected causes of uncertainty, well known in different fields of the production [4, 5]. It should also includes tools to detect minor issues that could have a major impact on the production, affecting not only the conformity of the products or services but also the overall budget. This follow-up of the production conformity is critical to classify the production at least at an acceptable level of specifications similar to what happens elsewhere in the industry.

Commonly, a manufacturing process is classified as "world class quality" when the average results (also designated arithmetic mean or mean) are "on target" with a "minimum variance," commonly referred as "6-sigma." Working with "minimum variance" is feasible uniquely when the process shows a reasonable degree of statistical control. The validation of the process of blood components' production is well established in blood establishments.

The establishment must prove that the production delivers compliant components not only in validation stage but also individually according to specifications and per lot. This is reported to show the requirements are continuously satisfied. The SPC is the standard method to control the production processes.

Theoretically, there are two measures of central tendency that indicate a failure in a process with an infinite number of samples: random error (entry 2.19 of [6]) and systematic error (entry 2.17 of [6]). Consequently, a theoretical variable from a normal distribution x with known σ and μ can be controlled. However, the σ and the μ are unknown, for what the variance and average of the results are estimated. When a normal distribution is unavailable, the data is normally transformed, or it is considered an attribute approach instead variables method (see 6). Any process has an expected error caused by the common/natural/expected sources of error. When it is identified that the error is higher than it is expected, it is assumed that special causes of error exist [7].

The traditional quality control approach has a short term strategy based on variance and out-of-specification results. The new way of thinking has a long-term strategy based on common and special causes. The relationship between the quality control and the manufacture is advisory in the traditional and cooperative in a new way. The responsibility for quality involves the quality control and quality assurance, or the staff cooperation in the production process to ensure compliance efficiently, respectively. Usually, it is related to the traditional approach a higher quality of outcomes with increased cost. The new approach is also recognized by the continuous satisfaction of high-quality requirements but with a significant decrease in the cost of products. Differently from the traditional concept which is focused principally on corrective actions, the new way is orientated to preventive measures/risk assessment [8].

The specification limits are selected according to what is mandatory, e.g., claims of blood components in the law. To fulfill the specification should be considered the primary goal. The SPC uses control charts to identify nonconforming lots or individual products, and capability indexes to classify the level of production. These charts include control limits informing if the process is operating properly, i.e., if the process operation assures a low probability to manufacture non-conforming products. These control limits are computed using error measurements arising from the principal sources of overall error such as human resources, critical equipment, and supplies. Process capability allows measuring the process ability to fulfill the production goals. A process could be in-control without meeting the specification or vice-versa. Note that only the samples are verified according to specifications, not according to control limits.

SPC is a process built on objective evidence to improve the delivery of conforming lots of products. Predominantly, this methodology is useful to improve the processes continuously. Therefore, it is proposed to decrease the variance, to control and report the stability of the processes, to follow-up the processes, to demonstrate the performance of the procedure, to previously detect for non-conformities about lots specifications, to document the process according to the law and other applicable requests.

This Chapter is related principally to SPC methodologies, including also a brief discussion about statistical sampling models such as practical cases in the blood components production. The reader is encouraged to apply the approaches using a dedicated SPC software such as Minitab® (Minitab Inc., State College, Pennsylvania, USA) or a spreadsheet software such as Excel® (Microsoft®, Redmond, Washington, USA).

2. Implementing the SPC in a Blood Establishment

A potential roadmap for the implementation should be developed. It is critical to identify what is mandatory and what actions are necessary to initialize the use of an SPC approach. It is defined the problem, the scope, and the stakeholders (interested parties) (entry 3.2.3 of [9]) identified. The staff in the production and the quality control laboratory should be coached and motivated, starting from the beginning of the implementation. Clearly, a management system should be established. The success of the implementation should be recognized, and the failures understood. According to the EDQM 2012 survey [10], there were 186 blood establishments in 33 European countries with an applied quality management system, and 51.9% fulfilling ISO 9001approach [11].

The trainer could take a real or theoretical examples for the problems. The staff should easily recognize this. It should be described in detail, focused on the stakeholders requirements. The persons that should be involved in the training should be evaluated (when is applicable) and the evaluation reported (entry 7.2 of [11]). The role of each of the individuals working with SPC activities is described. It is identified who has the responsibility for putting the data on the chart. Next to put the data in the graph, this person should be the first to verify if a statistical rule has been violated. It should also be identified who is accountable for the control chart. This individual has to verify on a lot basis that the operators fill in the chart correctly. This is the first person to be contacted if a statistical rule is violated. He is presenting the control chart to the process owner on a periodic basis (e.g., weekly), including observations, special causes, and actions. It is also identified who is consulted. These persons support the operating team in finding the root courses for special causes. Finally, it is identified who is informed. Usually, these individuals are the process owner and the leadership team. The staff should be currently informed about the state of the implementation (what is happening?). For example, using success and failure key performance indicators (KPI). Turning failure into success is a hard task, and avoiding failure is best but never possible.

The real world problems require the assurance of skilled and successfully trained personnel. It should be acknowledged that an employee with demonstrated competence in blood components specifications, basics of statistics and SPC requires a long-term formation to be capable of answering to the principal questions. So, when it is not possible to have some employee fulfilling these requirements, it should be hired a consultant with experience in SPC in the components production. In practice, it is known that is hard to have this employer. According to what is happening in blood establishments, it is suggested as a first step the support of a consultant and in a second phase to start the formation of someone that could be the responsible to maintain and develop the SPC methodology.

Implementing an SPC practice is a management decision. Senior management defines the criteria based on the voice of the customer (VoC) vs. voice of the business (VoB). VoC for blood components makes SPC recommend but not mandatory. VoB requires defining the critical product of business (high volume, high sales, high margin products) and the expected variatons. These changes are also studied associated with the cost per component. For example, using an analytical hierarchy process (AHP) scheme [12, 13]. The quality control, quality assurance and operating expenditure (OpEx) staff have the responsibility to create a list of the products and the criteria including specifications.

The identification of most sensitive parameters requires a careful review of blood components monitoring reports principally based on long-term data, e.g., the annual report checked for out of trend (OOT) observations. These reports should be studied by specialists and a failure mode, and effects risk analysis (FMEA) performed. Their recommendations should be proposed by the quality control, quality assurance and OpEx team and approved/rejected by the senior management.

3. UNDERSTANDING THE CAUSES OF VARIATION

The blood components production is a process $f(x)$ that has a repeatable value generating a sequence of activities transforming inputs x into reproducible outputs y, e.g., traceable whole blood and into traceable red cells component. The output of a process is associated to a variation, for what every process is affected by common causes of variation, sometimes described as "noise." The sources of this expected variation could be divided according to six categories: people, environment, methods, materials, measures, and equipment. Nonetheless, there is a specific component affecting the normal variation of the blood components: the biological variation of the testing parameters in humans beings, which cannot be corrected. This variation is not uniquely inter-individuals (between-subject) but also intra-individual (within-subject) [14]. Commonly, in the industry, the control of the input materials is an established practice. For example, this allows that a chemical material used in the production of a product has a nonsignificant impact in the normal error of the product. Otherwise, in a blood component, a primary source of normal error is derived from the biological variation. This limitation should be considered in the judgement of the capability of the process of production to accurate interpreation (see 7).

Special causes of variation occur when anytime something unexpected (special) occurs affecting the process variation. Finding the root-cause and removing the adverse effect or maintaining the positive effect is a chance for improvement. All processes gave a common cause of variation and, also occasionally a special cause of variation. Reducing the variation is a challenge that should be understood as possible, but it can never be removed. The special causes are identified using a root-cause analysis and differently from the common causes; those should be corrected, and corrective or preventive actions are used when applicable (entry 10.2 of [11]). The effort to find the root-cause for special causes increases with the complexity of the process. Control charts are the tools used to differentiate between common and special causes of variation. If the chance of 97.73% is established for a process, all the results do fall within "three standard deviations" $3s$. Due to practical reasons, this is defined as the Natural Process Limits where the data is between average

± 3s in an undisturbed practice. If any statistical rule is violated, then there is a variation arising from a special cause.

Wheeler (2009) suggests four classifications for any process according to its variation [15]:

a) Ideal state (no trouble) - The process demonstrates a common cause of variation and the product is 100% conforming;
b) Threshold state (product trouble) - The process exhibits a common cause of variation, but part of the product is non-conforming;
c) Brink of chaos (process trouble) - The process reveals a special cause of variation, but the product is 100% conforming;
d) State of chaos (double trouble) - The process exposes a special cause of variation, and part of the product is non-conforming.

It should be reflected the consequences if the measurement system is not capable, i.e., if the special causes are not detected in SPC or if there are a false rejection of lots due to inaccurate SPC (false alarms). Inaccurate evaluation of individual lots causes a waste in the budget. This could be directly related to additional testing of lots, erroneous rejection of lots, rework of lots, equipment inadequacy, high inventory or customer complaints.

The measurement system analysis is based on the evaluation of the total variance of the process and the measurement system. It is acknowledged as the sum of the squared measurement variance and the squared process variance. Thus, the process standard deviation is the square root of the difference between the total squared variance and the squared measurement variance. This approach is applied to long term checking.

4. SAMPLING

4.1. Sampling Method Applied to Production Lot

The most desirable in the manufacture of blood components should be to identify and measure each of the elements of the entire production. However, in the most of the situations, this is impracticable. Normally, the full production is distributed in production lots or lots. The sampling population is the lot, e.g., a weekly lot. The selection of an adequate rational subgrouping method is critical to a realistic sampling of the production. A rule of thumb is to use only subgroups with independently, identically, and normally distributed (IIND) data, whenever possible. In theory, the estimation of a subgrouping is commonly biased from the trueness of the production. However, the use of an adequate method assures a non-significant bias, i.e., the results are not significantly influenced. There are several sampling models such as simple random, systematic, and stratified sampling [16]. When the lot is long term, such a monthly lot, there is a significant risk to happen a special cause affecting a large number of distributed blood components. In this case, there is a significant hypothesis of non-conforming occurrences post-transfusion, such as ineffective transfusions and related clinical decisions. The lot should be adequate to the number of blood components manufactured and to the intended use. Systematic sampling or interval sampling could be applied to the production of blood components. At regular intervals (e.g., daily, weekly), a sampling is selected from a lot produced of each of the blood components type. This sampling method is used in a continuing series of lots of discrete products all supplied by a single blood establishment using one production process. When there is more than one manufacturer or process, the methodology should be applied independently in each one. It could be implemented to a unique measurable parameter on a continuous scale, normally over time.

Hypothetically the results in blood components could be biased or/and have a statistically major variance due to different posts of whole blood collection or due to different apheresis equipment. The laboratorian should verify statistically if these differences are significant. The significance of bias could be easily verified using the Student *t*-test between two groups. The analysis of variance (ANOVA) is used to check if there is a significant difference of the mean within and between at least in three groups (note: ANOVA is not used to test the difference between variances). The impact of variation could be explored using simply the two sample hypothesis *F*-test. If the null hypothesis H_0 is rejected, there is not a statistically significant difference between the mean at the 95.0% confidence level. A set of lots could be reunited in one single lot if the statistical differences are insignificant. The normality of the data distribution must be verified to apply theses statistical tools. Otherwise, the laboratorian should use non-parametric models.

4.2. Simple Random Sampling

The guide of the Council of Europe [3] recommends the number of samples equal to 1% with a minimum between four and 10 components (according to the tested analyte) of the monthly production per blood component. Mostly, this approach is applied in European blood establishments regularly without a statistical sampling method. The statistician immediately criticizes this method since the collection is not representative of the full production. This is a serious issue. For example, if the 1% is collected in the first days and the results are conforming to the specifications, these results cannot be statistically inferred to the full production and the risk cannot be known since a hypothesis test is not established. In this case, if the rest of the production is nonconforming, it is simply not identified since it is not sampled. Also, if an SPC method is applied to this sampling's results, it is useless due to the estimates are not based on a representative sampling. A suggested application of this approach could be the use of the simple random sampling of blood components. This method assures that each of the samples is selected randomly by probability, signifying that each of the blood components of a certain lot has the same chance to be chosen. Since it is the simplest probability of sampling methods, it does not require significant statistical skills to be computed. Using Excel®, a simple random sampling could be computed using the pseudo-random generator function RANDBETWEEN. Let consider the case where *plasma, fresh frozen* is tested before freezing. In this case, the EDQM guideline requires as minimum n = 1% of production, with a minimum of 10 units per month (entry Table 5D-1 (b) of [3]). If it is expected to produce during one month 100 plasmas, a minimum of 10 components is tested since 1% is equal to just one plasma. The days of the month are randomly selected. For example, = RANDBETWEEN(1,31) to select a random number between the 1st and 31st day. Therefore, the 10 samples are randomly selected, and the condition is repeated if the sample number is duplicate by pressing the keyboard F9. In this example, the sampling occurs in the 1st, 6th, 12th, 14th, 16th, 17th, 20th, 23th, 26th, and 28th day. In each day is collected one plasma. Again, it uses the simple sampling to select the plasma from each of the daily series. The plasmas are listed from 1 to +∞ according to the order of production. For example, =RANDBETWEEN(1,47) to choose a random number between the 1st and 47th plasma. In this case is the 12th plasma.

4.3. Sample Size

However, the question about the number of samples remains considering the EDQM requirements [3]. A simple approach to improve the "1% model" could be used. The sample size n in an infinite number of blood components normally distributed could be computed as follows:

$$n = \frac{z^2 s(1-s)}{E^2} \tag{1}$$

where z is selected from a z-score table considering a certain confidence interval, s is the standard deviation arising from the lot data, and E is the margin of error of the unknown mean of the production of a certain blood component. The margin of error expresses the chance of error per sampling. It represents the risk to the receptor of the blood component. Let consider a confidence interval of 95%, s equal to 0.01446 (n = 7), and E = 5%. It is determined as follows:

$$n = \frac{1.96^2(0.01446)(1-0.01446)}{0.05^2} = 21.9 = 22 \text{ (rounded up)}$$

Note that the sampling came from seven days, i.e., one week, so this is the case of a weekly lot. In this example, it is necessary to select randomly 22 samples during the seven days of the week. At least one sample is selected per sampling day. When the sample size of lots is stable (known N), it is possible to correct using a correction factor. However, this is not what systematically happens in a blood establishment. The blood establishment could consider that a certain number of samples is too large/costly. In this case, the confidence level should be carefully decreased, or the margin of error increased. Considering the previous case, but changing the confidence interval to 90% and the margin of error to 10%:

$$n = \frac{1.645^2(0.01446)(1-0.01446)}{0.1^2} = 3.9 = 4 \text{ (rounded up)}$$

Now only four samples are required. The blood establishment must verify if not only the minimum of 1% is satisfied but also the lowest number of samples request by the EDQM [3] or law. For example, if the lot is equal to

620 components, the confidence interval should increase and the margin of error decrease. It should be clearly known that SPC results can be applied only to 90% of a randomly selected number of a certain blood component. It should be recognized that till 10% of the certain blood component production could be nonconforming.

4.4. Sampling Based in the ISO 3951

The use ISO 3951-Part 1 includes sampling procedures for inspection by variables. Its approach is only applicable when is assumed a normal distribution of the measurements. Therefore, the normality is verified before sampling begins (entry 18.1 of [17]). Usually, it is checked in the previous validation of the production method per blood component. This happens using tests such as the D'Agostino-Pearson K^2 normality test (see 5.1) [18]. The ISO guideline is intended to determine a certain number of samples according to the size of a lot and the inspection level.

The sampling starts with the s-method and if the production process shows to have a long-term stability moves to the σ-method. The stability is understood not only as related to the statistical measures of central tendency, principally average measures but also to the systematical fulfillment of the individual requirements of each sample. s-method requires a larger number of samples since it is based on short-term data. Otherwise, σ-method is based in the long-term past of a stable process of production, requiring shorter samplings. Consequently, the cost per blood components produced is higher using s-method. The use of the σ-method since the beginning of a production represents a significant risk to accept or reject lots erroneously due to be less costly. Even considering that each sample is validated individually. It could be the starting method also when the s-method is not used, but there is favorable significant long-term evidence about the stability of the process (confident process). For example, testing the retrospective standard deviation. The selection between σ-method and s-method must be clearly demonstrated, i.e., it should be shown a long-term stable standard deviation if σ-method is selected (entry 11 of [17]).

ISO 3951-1 depends on the inspection level of the acceptance quality limit (AQL) defined as the "worst tolerable process fraction nonconforming when a continuing series of lots is submitted for acceptance sampling" (entry 3.6 of [17]). Usually, the inspection of sampling includes three models: normal, tightened, and reduced inspection. In this Chapter the inspection level is associated with the capability indexes as follows:

a) For each of the methods the inspection level chosen in the starting of the sampling plan is the normal level (level II);
b) The switch from normal to tightened inspection (level III) occurs when the inspection results show that the capability of the process is inadequate ($\hat{C}_{pk} < 1$);
c) The change from normal to reduced inspection (level I) happens when the capability of the process is systematically satisfactory ($\hat{C}_{pk} \geq 1.33$);
d) The switch from tightened to normal inspection occurs when the inspection results demonstrate that the capability of the process is continuously capable ($1 \leq \hat{C}_{pk} < 1.33$), and;
e) The change from reduced to normal inspection takes place when the capability of the process is capable ($1 \leq \hat{C}_{pk} < 1.33$) (see 7.1).

Table 1. Sample-size code letters for general inspection levels for inspection *s*-method

[%]

Lot size		I			II			III		
		Letter	Higher	Lower	Letter	Higher	Lower	Letter	Higher	Lower
2	8	B	100.0	37.5	B	100.0	37.5	B	100.0	37.5
9	15	B	33.3	20.0	B	33.3	20.0	C	44.4	26.7
16	25	B	18.8	12.0	C	25.0	16.0	D	37.5	24.0
26	50	C	11.5	6.0	D	23.1	12.0	E	34.6	18.0
51	90	C	5.9	3.3	E	17.6	10.0	F	25.5	14.4
91	150	D	3.3	2.0	F	14.3	8.7	G	19.8	12.0
151	280	F	4.0	2.1	G	11.9	6.4	H	16.6	8.9
281	500	F	2.1	1.2	H	8.9	5.0	J	12.5	7.0
501	1 200	G	1.8	0.8	J	7.0	2.9	K	10.0	4.2
1 201	3 200	H	1.1	0.4	K	4.2	1.6	L	5.8	2.2
3 201	10 000	J	0.6	0.2	L	2.2	0.7	M	3.0	1.0
10 001	35 000	K	0.2	0.1	M	0.9	0.3	N	1.2	0.4
35 001	150 000	L	0.1	0.0	N	0.4	0.1	P	0.5	0.1
150 001	500 000	M	0.0	0.0	P	0.1	0.0	Q	0.1	0.0
500 000	$+\infty$	N	0.0	0.0	Q	0.0	0.0	R	0.1	0.1

Table 2. Sample-size code letters for general inspection levels for inspection σ-method

[%]

Lot size		I			II			III		
		Letter	Higher	Lower	Letter	Higher	Lower	Letter	Higher	Lower
2	8	B	100.0	25.0	B	100.0	25.0	B	100.0	25.0
9	15	B	22.2	13.3	B	22.2	13.3	C	33.3	20.0
16	25	B	12.5	8.0	C	18.8	12.0	D	25.0	16.0
26	50	C	7.7	4.0	D	15.4	8.0	E	23.1	12.0
51	90	C	3.9	2.2	E	11.8	6.7	F	15.7	8.9
91	150	D	2.2	1.3	F	8.8	5.3	G	11.0	6.7
151	280	F	2.6	1.4	G	6.6	3.6	H	7.9	4.3
281	500	F	1.4	0.8	H	4.3	2.4	J	5.3	3.0
501	1 200	G	1.2	0.5	J	3.0	1.3	K	3.6	1.5
1 201	3 200	H	0.7	0.3	K	1.5	0.6	L	1.7	0.7
3 201	10 000	J	0.3	0.1	L	0.7	0.2	M	0.8	0.3
10 001	35 000	K	0.1	0.0	M	0.2	0.1	N	0.3	0.1
35 001	150 000	L	0.0	0.0	N	0.1	0.0	P	0.1	0.0
150 001	500 000	M	0.0	0.0	P	0.0	0.0	Q	0.0	0.0
500 000	+∞	N	0.0	0.0	Q	0.0	0.0	R	0.0	0.0

Table 3. Sample sizes for sample-size code letters and inspection method

	s-method		σ-method	
Letter	Normal and tightened inspection	Reduced inspection	Normal and tightened inspection	Reduced inspection
B	3	3	2	2
C	4	3	3	2
D	6	3	4	2
E	9	4	6	3
F	13	6	8	4
G	18	9	10	6
H	25	13	12	8
J	35	18	15	10
K	50	25	18	12
L	70	35	21	15
M	95	50	25	18
N	125	70	32	21
P	160	95	40	25
Q	200	125	50	32
R	250	160	65	40

The appropriate sample size is determined using a set of tables. Let consider a daily lot of *red cells, leucocyte depleted in additive solution* components with $N = 97$. The number of samples n is determined as follows:

a) The lot size is selected choosing the letter of normal inspection level in the s-method (Table 1), i.e., letter F in level II (if it is starting using the σ-method Table 2 is applied), and;
b) Use Table 3 to select the n according to the normal inspection level in the s-method, which is equal to 13 samples.

The 13 *red cells, leucocyte depleted in additive solution* components could be identified using a simple random generator (see 4.2). For further details about the use of the ISO 3951 approach, please refer to [17].

The ISO 3951-1 approach has several advantages over the use of uniquely the simple random sampling. Principally, because it considers the retrospective data before starting a sampling plan and due to enabling the user to change the sampling plan level according to the capability index. Also, the samples size is pre-determined, making it simpler to the user.

5. The Data Reliability

5.1. Detection of Outliers

An outlier is an observation that seems to diverge noticeably from others in a sampling [19]. A single outlier could increase the variation, changing the average and could even alter the acceptance of a lot. Outliers should be removed to avoid the risk to affect the statistical analysis of the sampling. Often the "common-sense" judgment of the analyst (or pair of analysts) is used. However, human error influences the decision, for what could be risky to samplings when large n is verified. It is recommended to consider the "common-sense" with statistical tests such as the Grubbs test to detect a single outlier [20]. When an outlier is removed it is reported the basis of the decision. If the result is a true result, it should not be treated equally, e.g., a true result when is higher than $3s$ cannot be handled as an outlier. When it is suspected more than one outlier, it could be used the Generalized Extreme Studentized Deviate (ESD) test [21] or the Tukey test [22]. For example, considering the hematocrit results (ratio) in a normally distributed sampling consisting of 90 *red cells, leucocyte depleted in additive solution* components. In this case the maximum and minimum values are 0.56 and 0.63. The normality is tested using three tests in MedCalc® software (Medcalc Software bvba, Ostend, Belgium): the *p*-value is equal or higher than to 0.05 to the Grubbs double-sided and ESD tests for what none outlier is identified which is also verified by the Tukey's test. The *p*-value value is interpreted as the chance of a sample in this rational subgroup to be an outlier is not significant at the 0.05 significance level.

5.2. The Importance of the Normal Distribution

The normality should be verified previously to the starting sampling. The D'Agostino-Pearson K^2 normality test is a statistical inference technique designed to test that the underlying distribution of a random variable is normally distributed [18]. For testing that the blood components production is normally distributed, the skewness and kurtosis statistics are combined in the D'Agostino-Pearson K^2 test outcome. The test first computes the skewness and kurtosis to quantify how far from the normal distribution is regarding the asymmetry and shape. It is calculated how far each of these values differs from the value expected for a normal distribution, computing a single *p*-value from the sum of these differences. The test should be applied to a number of samples higher than 20. Using the same data than in the example before in MedCalc®, the *p*-value is equal or higher than 0.05 to the D'Agostino-Pearson test ($p = 0.5099$) whereby the normality distribution is not rejected.

6. Control Charts

6.1. Types of Control Charts

There are a set of control charts that are selected according to factors such as the number of samples, data distribution, expiration date of the products, use of destructive testing methods, and the budget. They could be divided in variable or attributes charts. The variable charts require numerical measurement. For example, the hematocrit is a variable of *red cells, leucocyte depleted in additive solution* components. These charts commonly require monitoring the average and the variability of the process. Certain variable charts also depend on the data distribution. One of the misunderstandings of the use of variables is to consider that many samples with results out-of-specifications are statistically rejected. This case is also a misunderstood of the SPC goal. The use of quality control charts with variables able to show the state of the process such as the quality control rules in each bath in real time. They cannot be applied when a parameter of a product is not expressed in a numerical quantity, or the data distribution is inapplicable to a specific model. For example, leucocytes have a logarithmic distribution, therefore, cannot be used in charts requiring normally distributed data. One option is to transform the data, and another is to use attributes charts. These charts use the number of nominal observations (entry 1.30 of [6]), e.g., the number of nonconforming results or a number of defects. Its use should be a secondary option since the information given using attributes is minimal when compared to the use of numerical measurements. The attribute charts are not so useful to determine the special causes since it is uniquely known the number or ratio of results rejected in sampling. Also the risk to accept non-conforming products is considerably higher, since the rules are verified commonly in a large number of samples (e.g., 150 blood components), for what the control is retrospective. They have advantages, such as the cheaper cost of inspection since it requires a shorter number of samples and a simpler approach. The concept is also easier to understand by the laboratorian.

There are many different control charts to be used in SPC, including charts for special purposes, such as the Wear-and-Tear-Control Charts [23] and the Multi-Variate-Control Charts [24]. This Chapter is orientated to charts suitable to monitor the quality of the blood components production:

a) Individual value and moving average chart,
b) Average and range chart,
c) Average and standard deviation chart, and;
d) Control charts for attributes.

All the charts and calculus in following examples are computed with Minitab® software.

6.2. Control Charts for Variables

6.2.1. Individual and Moving Ranges Charts

The individual and moving range charts (x-$\overline{R}$ charts) are intended to verify significant changes of random and systematic error components in $\overline{R}$-chart and x-chart, respectively. The individual sample results chart is used when a number of products is considerably small. Also, when is required that the products are fully tested instead sampled. The x-chart evaluates the systematic variation over time ("long-term" variation). The average of the individual results is similar to the mean of the entire production when the data is normally distributed. Theoretically, the standard deviation determination using cumulative results from the accepted lot is complementary to the moving average. However, in the production of blood components, the number of samples per rationale subgrouping is continuously equal or less than 10, thus the moving range is used instead the "moving standard deviation." The $\bar{R}$-chart evaluates the "short-term" variation in ranges between successive samples, complementing the x-chart estimate.

The mathematical model expressing the moving average is:

$$MR_i = |x_i - x_{i-1}| \tag{2}$$

where x_i is the observation i, and x_{i-1} is the previous observation.

The center line of the x-chart is the outcome of the average of the individual results in-control conditions. It is calculated as follows:

$$\bar{x} = \frac{\sum_{i=1}^{n} x_i}{n} \tag{3}$$

where x_i is the observation i, $i = 1,\ldots,n$, and n is the number of observations.

The control limits are determined using the following mathematical models:

$$UCL_x = \bar{x} + 3\frac{\overline{MR}}{d_2} \tag{4}$$

$$LCL_x = \bar{x} - 3\frac{\overline{MR}}{d_2} \tag{5}$$

where $\bar{x}$ is the average of the individual results, $\overline{MR}$ is the average of moving ranges, see Equation (6), and d_2 is the constant for a number of samplings m (see Table 4 for sigma estimate).

Table 4. Table of control charts constants

	$\bar{x}$-chart constants		R-chart constants		For sigma estimate	s-chart constants		
Sample size m	A_2	A_3	D_3	D_4	d_2	B_3	B_4	C_4
2	1.880	2.659	0	3.267	1.128	0	3.267	0.7979
3	1.023	1.954	0	2.574	1.693	0	2.568	0.8862
4	0.729	1.628	0	2.282	2.059	0	2.266	0.9213
5	0.577	1.427	0	2.114	2.326	0	2.089	0.9400
6	0.483	1.287	0	2.004	2.534	0.030	1.970	0.9515
7	0.419	1.182	0.076	1.924	2.704	0.118	1.882	0.9594
8	0.373	1.099	0.136	1.864	2.847	0.185	1.815	0.9650
9	0.337	1.032	0.184	1.816	2.970	0.239	1.761	0.9693
10	0.308	0.975	0.223	1.777	3.078	0.284	1.716	0.9727
11	0.285	0.927	0.256	1.774	3.173	0.321	1.679	0.9754
12	0.266	0.886	0.284	1.716	3.258	0.354	1.646	0.9776
13	0.249	0.850	0.308	1.692	3.336	0.382	1.618	0.9794
14	0.235	0.817	0.329	1.671	3.407	0.406	1.594	0.9810
15	0.223	0.789	0.348	1.652	3.472	0.428	1.572	0.9823
16	0.212	0.763	0.364	1.636	3.532	0.448	1.552	0.9835
17	0.203	0.739	0.379	1.621	3.588	0.466	1.534	0.9845
18	0.194	0.718	0.392	1.608	3.640	0.482	1.518	0.9854
19	0.187	0.698	0.404	1.596	3.689	0.497	1.503	0.9862
20	0.180	0.680	0.414	1.586	3.735	0.510	1.490	0.9869
21	0.173	0.663	0.425	1.575	3.778	0.523	1.477	0.9876
22	0.167	0.647	0.434	1.566	3.819	0.534	1.466	0.9882
23	0.162	0.633	0.443	1.557	3.858	0.545	1.455	0.9887
24	0.157	0.619	0.452	1.548	3.895	0.555	1.445	0.9892
25	0.153	0.606	0.459	1.541	3.9	0.565	1.435	0.9896

The center line of the $\bar{R}$-chart is the outcome of the average of the moving ranges in-control conditions, determined according to the model:

$$\overline{MR} = \frac{\sum_{i=1}^{n} MR_i}{n-1} \tag{6}$$

where for MR_i see Equation (2), and for n individual values there are n-1 ranges. Accordingly, $\overline{MR}$ expresses the average of the ranges in a number of lots during a given period. Only the combination of the moving average and the moving range permit to understand the overall level of confidence in the production considering individual results, due to their complementarity.

The control limits in the $\overline{R}$ -chart are calculated as follows:

$$UCL_x = D_4\overline{MR} \tag{7}$$

$$LCL_x = 0$$

where for $\overline{MR}$ see Equation (6), and D_4 is the constant for a number of samplings m (see Table 4 for R-chart constants).

The calculation of the control limits should be based on 20 to 30 data points in reproducibility conditions. The use of a shorter sampling or repeatability conditions makes the estimates unrealistic (unaccurate). This causes the incorrect use of the statistical rules (i.e., “false alarms”) since the control limits are erroneously short. If there are more than 30 data points, there is a high chance that special causes affect the process, and the control limits are wider than they should be.

The control limit should be calculated (updated) with every new data point. However, the calculating conditions of control limits should be carefully checked. Results caused by special causes cannot be used to update limits. Control limits are recalculated if the change is positive, the root-cause is identified, there is assurance that the modification is going to be permanent, and at least 20 samples confirm the new process. All these four rules are applied simultaneously.

After the establishment of a chart, each new point is checked to very if any rule is violated. If a statistical rule is violated, there is a special cause of variation (entry 6.4 of [25]).

Let consider the hematocrit results (ratio) in a sampling with 30 *red cells, leucocyte depleted in additive solution* components. This collection is the first 30 components manufactured in a small blood establishment where the full production is tested. Figure 1 shows the x-$\overline{R}$ charts. This case data is displayed in Table 5. Equation (3) is applied to determine the center line and Equations (4) and (5) to determine the x-chart control limits as follows:

$$\overline{x} = \frac{\sum_{i=1}^{30} x_i}{30} = \frac{18.17}{30} = 0.61 \text{, } UCL_x = 0.60567 + 3\frac{0.01586}{1.128} = 0.65 \text{,}$$

and $LCL_x = 0.56$

Equation (6) is applied to determine the center line and Equations (7) to determine the $\overline{R}$-chart control limits as follows:

$$\overline{MR} = \frac{\sum_{i=1}^{30} MR_i}{29} = \frac{0.46}{29} = 0.02\text{, } UCL_x = 3.267(0.01586) = 0.05\text{, and } LCL_x = 0$$

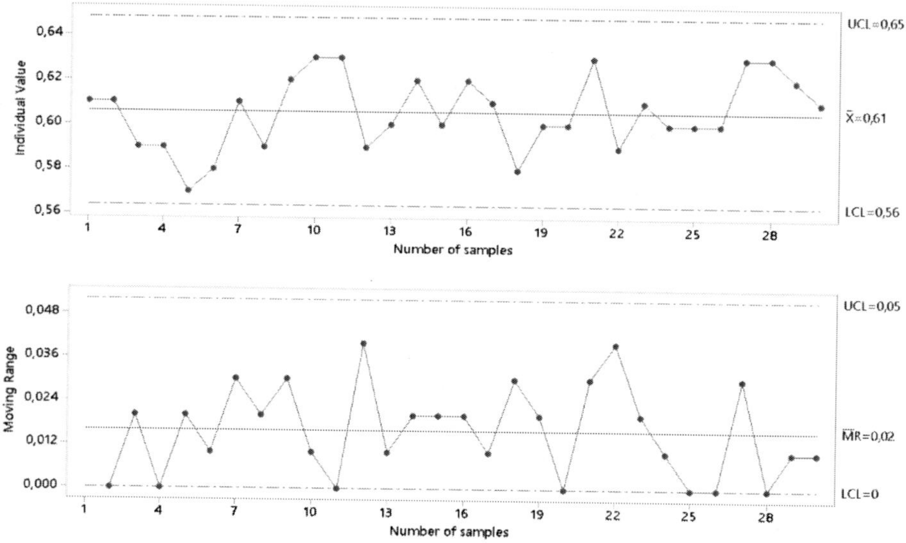

Figure 1. x-$\overline{R}$ charts for the control of hematocrit (ratio) in a series of individual results.

Table 5. Individual *red cells, leucocyte depleted in additive solution* components

No.	Hematocrit (ratio) x	*MR*	No.	Hematocrit (ratio) x	*MR*	No.	Hematocrit (ratio) x	*MR*
1	0.61	0	11	0.63	0	21	0.63	0.03
2	0.61	0	12	0.59	0.04	22	0.59	0.04
3	0.59	0.02	13	0.60	0.01	23	0.61	0.02
4	0.59	0	14	0.62	0.02	24	0.60	0.01
5	0.57	0.02	15	0.60	0.02	25	0.60	0
6	0.58	0.01	16	0.62	0.02	26	0.60	0
7	0.61	0.03	17	0.61	0.01	27	0.63	0.03
8	0.59	0.02	18	0.58	0.03	28	0.63	0
9	0.62	0.03	19	0.60	0.02	29	0.62	0.01
10	0.63	0.01	20	0.60	0	30	0.61	0.01
							$\overline{x} = 0.61$	$\overline{MR} = 0.02$

6.2.2. Average and Range Charts

The average and range charts ($\bar{x}$-R charts) are used when there are frequently lots/sampling (e.g., daily lots). The sampling is collected according to a statistical sampling model (see 4). The observations per sampling are computed to determine the average, range, to plot these points to verify if the lot is in or out-of-control. Whenever possible, the sampling should not happen retrospectively to decrease the risk to distribute non-complaint blood components. Since it is useful do identify the variation between lots, the $\bar{x}$-R charts are a useful for this purpose. The $\bar{x}$-chart is intended to verify the variation between lots (process changes). The R chart verifies the variation within a lot (short-term variation).

The average is a measure of central tendency. It is the sum of a group of numbers divided by the number of numbers in the group, see Equation (3).

The range is the difference between the largest and smallest of the values, in the case of the SPC is the difference between two consecutive measurements as follows:

$$R = x_{\max} - x_{\min} \tag{8}$$

where $x_{\max}$ is the maximum and $x_{\min}$ is the minimum value of sampling. Once again, outliers critically influence this determination. It is a model that is used instead of variance when the sampling is equal or less than 10 since it expresses a more realistic estimate of the random error. The range through a lot should not be used to assess the variance of a parameter determined between lots since within lot are not equal from between lot statistics.

Erroneous extreme numbers influence also the average, for what it could be unrealistic estimated when outliers occur and are not detected. The random error influences the accuracy of average since lower variances increase the chance of the average result to occur. Otherwise, larger random error signifies that the average has a low chance to happen. Bias also influences it, which quantifies the distant between the average and the reference value (an approximation to the true). Averages with significant bias could be corrected.

To determine the center line of the $\bar{x}$ chart it is required the calculus of the average of the sampling using the model equation:

$$\bar{\bar{x}} = \frac{\sum_{i=1}^{m} \bar{x}_i}{m} \tag{9}$$

where for x see Equation (3), x_i is the observation i, $i = 1,\ldots,m$, and m is the number of samplings.

The average control limits, the upper control limit $UCL_{\bar{x}}$ and the lower control limit $LCL_{\bar{x}}$, are computing as follows:

$$UCL_{\bar{x}} = \bar{\bar{x}} + A_2\bar{R} \tag{10}$$

$$LCL_{\bar{x}} = \bar{\bar{x}} - A_2\bar{R} \tag{11}$$

where $\bar{\bar{x}}$ is the average of the sample means, A_2 is the $\bar{x}$**-chart** constant for a number of samplings m (see Table 4), and for $\bar{R}$ is the average of ranges. These control limits are equivalent to three-sigma control, α = 0.0027, and the identical is considered in the R chart.

To determine the center line of the R-chart is determined the average range of the samples using the model:

$$\bar{R} = \frac{\sum_{i=1}^{n} R_i}{m-1} \tag{12}$$

where R_i is the range i, $i = 1,\ldots,m$, and m is the number of samplings. To emphasize that R is related to the sigma regarding a constant (depending on m) listed in statistical tables, sigma is equal to the $\bar{R}$ divided by the constant d_2 (see Table 4 for sigma estimate). Consequently, when the R-chart is in-control, sigma is computed using the unbiased estimator:

$$\hat{\sigma} = \frac{\bar{R}}{d_2} \tag{13}$$

where $\bar{R}$ is the average of ranges and d_2 is the constant for sigma estimate for a number of samplings m (see Table 4).

The R chart control limits, the upper control limit UCL_R and the lower control limit LCL_R, are computed using the following models:

$$UCL_R = D_4\bar{R} \tag{14}$$

where $\bar{R}_2$ is the average of ranges and D_4 is the R-chart constant for a number of samplings m (see Table 4).

The LCL range is determined using the model:

$$LCL_R = D_3\bar{R} \tag{15}$$

where $\bar{R}$ is the average of ranges and D_3 is the R-chart constant for a number of samplings m (see Table 4).

In the development of Equations (11) and (12) the σ_R substitutes the $\bar{R}$ component in the determination of the R-chart control limits to enhance the realism of estimates. Therefore, the model equations are rewritten considering A_2 equal to the division of three by the product of the multiplication of d_2 (see Table 4 for sigma estimate) by the square root of m:

$$UCL_{\bar{x}} = \bar{\bar{x}} + \frac{3}{d_2\sqrt{n}}\bar{R} \tag{16}$$

$$LCL_{\bar{x}} = \bar{\bar{x}} - \frac{3}{d_2\sqrt{n}}\bar{R} \tag{17}$$

The development of Equations (14) and (15) it is assumed that the standard deviation of $R\,\hat{\sigma}_R$ is the product of the multiplication of d_3 by $\hat{\sigma}$, D_4 (see Table 4 for R-chart constants) is equal to the sum of one with the product of the multiplication of three by the result of the division of d_3 by d_2 (see Table 4 for sigma estimate). D_3 (see Table 4 for R-chart constants) is the difference between one and the product of the multiplication of three by the result of the division of d_3 by d_2 as follows:

$$UCL_R = \bar{R} + 3d_3\frac{\bar{R}}{d_2} \tag{18}$$

$$LCL_R = \bar{R} - 3d_3\frac{\bar{R}}{d_2} \tag{19}$$

A rule of the thumb in $\bar{x}$-R charts is if the R-chart is out-of-control the $\bar{x}$-chart control limits cannot be a reliable estimate, for what they are unacceptable. Note that the R-chart has LCL equal to zero when the sampling size is equal or less than six (entry 6.2 of [25]).

Considering the hematocrit results (ratio) in a 30 lots sampling with a constant sampling equal to three *red cells, leucocyte depleted in additive solution* components. This is a collection of a blood establishment where the production per daily lot does not significantly vary. Figure 2 shows the $\bar{x}$-R charts. Table 6 lists the data of this case. Equation (9) is applied to determine the center line, and Equations (10) and (11) to the control limits of the $\bar{x}$-chart as follows:

$$\bar{\bar{x}} = \frac{\sum_{i=1}^{30} \bar{x}_i}{30} = \frac{18.02}{30} = 0.60\ ,\ UCL_{\bar{x}} = 0.60067 + 1.023 \cdot 0.02733 = 0.63\ ,$$

and $LCL_{\bar{x}} = 0.57$

Equation (12) is applied to determine the center line and Equations (14) and (15) to the control limits of the R-chart as follows:

$$\bar{R} = \frac{\sum_{i=1}^{30} R_i}{30} = \frac{0.82}{30} = 0.03\ ,\ UCL_R = 2.574 \cdot 0.02733 = 0.07\ ,$$

and $LCL_R = 0 \cdot 0.02733 = 0$

6.2.3. Average and Standard Deviation Charts

The creation and operation of average and standard deviation charts ($\bar{x}$-s charts) are close to those of $\bar{x}$-R charts. The difference is that for each one it is computed the sample average and the sample standard deviation. The $\bar{x}$-R charts are commonly preferred to the $\bar{x}$-s charts when are using fixed samplings. $\bar{x}$-s charts are applied to variable sampling, where the $\bar{x}$-R charts cannot be applied. The $\bar{x}$-R charts are generally not used in this situation since they lead to a changing center line on the R chart. In the condition with variable selection, it is used a weighted average method to calculate the center lines of both charts.

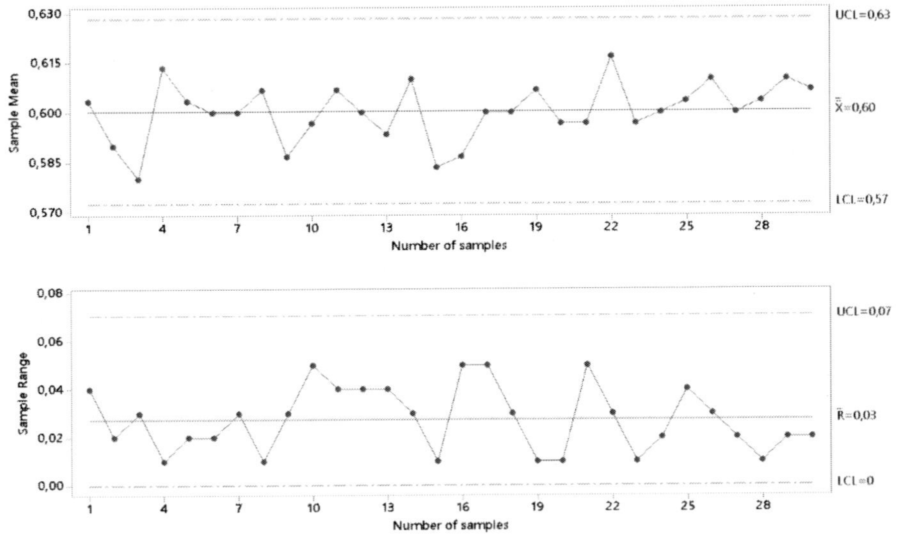

Figure 2. $\overline{x}$-R charts for the control of hematocrit (ratio) in a series of rational subgroups with a constant number of samples.

Table 6. Constant sampling of *red cells, leucocyte depleted in additive solution* components

	Observations						Observations				
No.	n_1	n_2	n_3	$\overline{x}_i$	R_i	No.	n_1	n_2	n_3	$\overline{x}_i$	R_i
1	0.62	0.58	0.61	0.6	0.04	16	0.59	0.56	0.61	0.59	0.05
2	0.58	0.60	0.59	0.59	0.02	17	0.63	0.58	0.59	0.6	0.05
3	0.56	0.59	0.59	0.58	0.03	18	0.61	0.58	0.61	0.6	0.03
4	0.61	0.61	0.62	0.61	0.01	19	0.61	0.61	0.60	0.61	0.01
5	0.61	0.59	0.61	0.6	0.02	20	0.60	0.60	0.59	0.6	0.01
6	0.60	0.61	0.59	0.6	0.02	21	0.62	0.57	0.60	0.6	0.05
7	0.62	0.59	0.59	0.6	0.03	22	0.60	0.63	0.62	0.62	0.03
8	0.60	0.61	0.61	0.61	0.01	23	0.60	0.60	0.59	0.6	0.01
9	0.57	0.60	0.59	0.59	0.03	24	0.60	0.59	0.61	0.6	0.02
10	0.57	0.62	0.60	0.6	0.05	25	0.61	0.58	0.62	0.6	0.04
11	0.59	0.60	0.63	0.61	0.04	26	0.63	0.60	0.60	0.61	0.03
12	0.58	0.60	0.62	0.6	0.04	27	0.60	0.59	0.61	0.6	0.02
13	0.57	0.60	0.61	0.59	0.04	28	0.61	0.60	0.60	0.6	0.01
14	0.60	0.60	0.63	0.61	0.03	29	0.62	0.60	0.61	0.61	0.02
15	0.58	0.58	0.59	0.58	0.01	30	0.60	0.60	0.62	0.61	0.02
								$\sum \overline{x}_i = 18.02$		$\sum R_i = 0.82$	
								$\overline{\overline{x}} = 0.60$		$\overline{R} = 0.03$	

To determine the center line of the $\bar{x}$-chart when sampling is variable it is calculated the average of the sampling using the model equation:

$$\bar{\bar{x}} = \frac{\sum_{i=1}^{m} n_i \bar{x}_i}{\sum_{i=1}^{m} n_i} \quad (20)$$

where $\bar{x}_i$ is the average i, $i = 1,\ldots,m$, m is the number of samplings, and n_i is the number of averages.

Although the variance is an unbiased estimator of sigma, the standard deviation is a biased estimator, for what a correction factor as a function of m is found in Table 4 (s-chart constants). The average control limits, the upper control limit $UCL_{\bar{x}}$, and the lower control limit $LCL_{\bar{x}}$, are computed using the following models for an unbiased estimate:

$$UCL_{\bar{x}} = \bar{\bar{x}} + A_3\bar{s} \quad (21)$$

$$LCL_{\bar{x}} = \bar{\bar{x}} - A_3\bar{s} \quad (22)$$

where $\bar{\bar{x}}$ is the average of the sample means, A_3 is the $\bar{x}$-chart constant for a number of samplings m (see Table 4), and;

The constant A_3 is according to the sample size of each rational subgroup.

To determine the center line of the s-chart is determined the average range of the samples using the model:

$$\bar{s} = \sqrt{\frac{\sum_{i=1}^{m} (n_i - 1)s_i^2}{\sum_{i=1}^{m} n_i - m}} \quad (23)$$

where s_i is the standard deviation i, $i = 1,\ldots,m$, m is the number of samplings, and n_i is the number of standard deviations.

The average control limits, the upper control limit UCL_s, and the lower control limit LCL_s, are computed in the same situation using the following models for an unbiased estimate:

$$UCL_s = B_4\bar{s} \tag{24}$$

where B_4 is the $\bar{x}$-chart constant for a number of samplings m (see Table 4), and $\bar{s}$ is the average of standard deviation.

$$LCL_s = B_3\bar{s} \tag{25}$$

where B_3 is the $\bar{x}$-chart constant for a number of samplings m (see Table 4), and $\bar{s}$ is the average of the standard deviation. The constant B_3 and B_4 is according to the sample size of each subgroup (entry 6.3 of [25]).

Let consider the hematocrit results (ratio) in a sampling with 30 lots with a variable number of samples per sampling of *red cells, leucocyte depleted in additive solution* components. This rational subgroup is from a blood establishment that manufactures a daily lot where the sampling is according to the significantly different number of blood components produced. Differently from the previous charts, in $\bar{x}$-s charts with a variable number of samples, the control limits are determined per rational subgroup. Figure 3 shows the $\bar{x}$-s charts. Table 7 displays this cases' data. Equation (20) expresses the center line and Equations (21) and (22) the control limits of $\bar{x}$-chart as follows:

$$\bar{\bar{x}} = \frac{\sum_{i=1}^{30} n_i\bar{x}_i}{\sum_{i=1}^{30} n_i} = \frac{5(0.596)+4(0.5950)+\cdots+4(0.6025)}{5+4+\cdots+4} = \frac{72.68}{121} = 0.60,$$

$UCL_{\bar{x}} = 0.60066 + A_3\bar{s}$, and $LCL_{\bar{x}} = \bar{\bar{x}} - A_3\bar{s}$ (note: for the first sample n_1, $m = 5$)

Equation (23) compute the center line and Equations (24) and (25) the control limits of R-chart as follows:

$$\bar{s} = \sqrt{\frac{\sum_{i=1}^{30}(n_i-1)s_i^2}{\sum_{i=1}^{30} n_i - 30}} = \sqrt{\frac{4(0.00043)+3(0.00017)+\cdots+3(0.00016)}{5+4+\cdots 4-30}} = \sqrt{\frac{0.02226}{91}} = 0.02,$$

$UCL_s = 2.089(0.01564) = 0.03$, and $LCL_s = 0(0.01564) = 0$

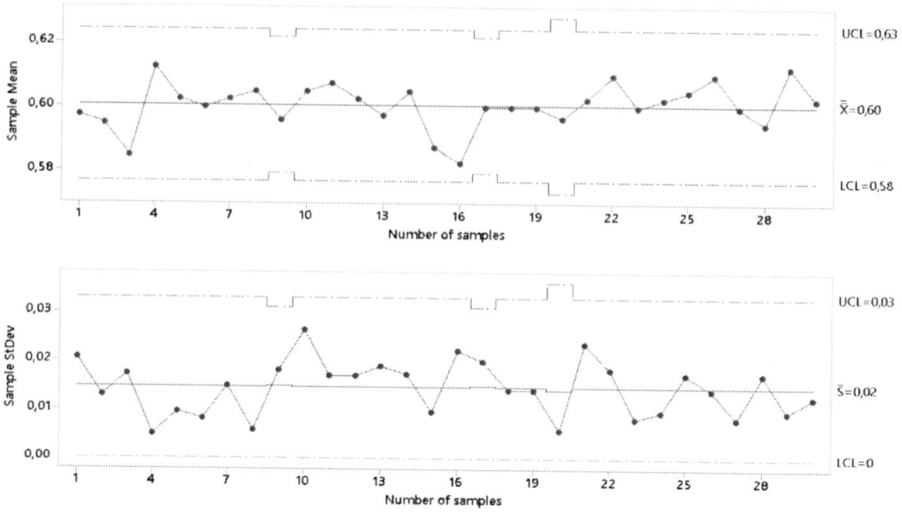

Figure 3. $\overline{x}$-s charts for the control of hematocrit (ratio) in a series of rational subgroups with a variable number of samples.

6.2.4. Interpreting Control Charts

Special patterns could be observed in charts. A result outside the control limits is an indicator of non-randomness. However, other unnatural patterns are possible to happen including patterns with results within control limits. For example, a cyclic pattern with a periodic signal, a mixtures pattern with two or more sources, shifts indicating an abrupt change, trends representing a gradual change, and stratification indicating the variability is too minor (entry 6.2.4 of [25]). There are available different sets of decision rules that could be applied to detect these examples of special patterns. The use of inadequate rules could lead to an increase of the false alarms. Statistical rules are used to test for the special cause of variation. Despite the use of rules, a set of conditions could interfere in the outcomes. So, the reading is verified if it is accurate, e.g., verifying the reported validation of the test and the internal quality control, and if the result is not an outlier.

Usually, 20 to 30 results are required to establish control limits. These results are conforming according to the specifications. To classify points out-of-control when control limits are not defined is a challenge to the quality control decision maker. Typically, when the out-of-control results are explained, they are rejected from the calculation of control limits and central line. If they cannot be understood they should not be rejected. It is expected to have close to one false alarm per 370 samples for 3σ control limits. Again, the control limits should not be easily reviewed.

Table 7. Variable sampling of *red cells, leucocyte depleted in additive solution* components

	Observations								Observations						
No.	n_1	n_2	n_3	n_3	n_4	$\overline{x}_i$	s_i	No.	n_1	n_2	n_3	n_3	n_4	$\overline{x}_i$	s_i
1	0.62	0.58	0.61	0.58	-	0.5975	0.02062	1	0.62	0.58	0.61	0.58	-	0.5975	0.02062
2	0.58	0.60	0.59	0.61	-	0.595	0.01291	17	0.63	0.58	0.59	0.59	0.61	0.6	0.02
3	0.56	0.59	0.59	0.60	-	0.585	0.01732	18	0.61	0.58	0.61	0.60	-	0.6	0.01414
4	0.61	0.61	0.62	0.61	-	0.6125	0.005	19	0.61	0.61	0.60	0.58	-	0.6	0.01414
5	0.61	0.59	0.61	0.60	-	0.6025	0.00957	20	0.60	0.60	0.59	-	-	0.5967	0.00577
6	0.60	0.61	0.59	0.60	-	0.6	0.00817	21	0.62	0.57	0.60	0.62	-	0.6025	0.02363
7	0.62	0.59	0.59	0.61	-	0.6025	0.015	22	0.60	0.63	0.62	0.59	-	0.61	0.01826
8	0.60	0.61	0.61	0.60	-	0.605	0.00577	23	0.60	0.60	0.59	0.61	-	0.6	0.00817
9	0.57	0.60	0.59	0.60	0.62	0.596	0.01817	24	0.60	0.59	0.61	0.61	-	0.6025	0.00957
10	0.57	0.62	0.60	0.63	-	0.605	0.02646	25	0.61	0.58	0.62	0.61	-	0.605	0.01732
11	0.59	0.60	0.63	0.61	-	0.6075	0.01708	26	0.63	0.60	0.60	0.61	-	0.61	0.01414
12	0.58	0.60	0.62	0.61	-	0.6025	0.01708	27	0.60	0.59	0.61	0.60	-	0.6	0.00817
13	0.57	0.60	0.61	0.61	-	0.5975	0.01893	28	0.61	0.60	0.60	0.57	-	0.595	0.01732
14	0.60	0.60	0.63	0.59	-	0.605	0.01732	29	0.62	0.60	0.61	0.62	-	0.6125	0.00957
15	0.58	0.58	0.59	0.60	-	0.5875	0.00957	30	0.60	0.60	0.62	0.59	-	0.6025	0.01258
														$\sum \overline{x}_i = 18.02017$	$\sum s_i = 0.43393$
														$\overline{\overline{x}} = 0.60$	$\overline{s} = 0.02$

Another rule of the thumb is that the $\overline{x}$-chart is only valid if the variability in the R or $\overline{R}$-chart is normal, such as is related in the s-chart and the $\overline{x}$-chart. Therefore, the R or $\overline{R}$-chart and the s-chart are analyzed using decision rules first. The user cannot accept results according to the $\overline{x}$-chart if one of the R, $\overline{R}$-chart or the s-chart is out-of-control. In this case, the estimates of average are unrealistic.

The basic condition that is applied is that one or more points are not expected to be outside of the control limits in normal condition. However, it does not permit to detect any other unnatural pattern. A well-established set of rules is the Western Electric rules that are applied in the industry since 1956 [7], and are intended to detect a series of unnatural patterns (increasing the sensitivity of detection). Three zones are considered in the use of these rules: A zone is between the 2σ and the 3σ limit, B zone is between the 2σ and 1σ limit, and C zone is between the 1σ and the center line.

The Western Electric rules:
Rule 1. One point outside of the control limit 3σ;
Rule 2. Two points out of three are more than 2σ from the center line;
Rule 3. Four points out of five are more than 1σ from the center line;
Rule 4. Nine points on one side of the center line;
Rule 5. Six points increasing or decreasing;
Rule 6. Fourteen points alternating up and down, and;
Rule 7. Fifteen points on either side in center line ± 1σ.

The first four rules are known as the "zone rules," and are accepted as the most important of the Western Electric set. The four rules identify the process instability. The probability of each one of the "zone rules" to occur is probably the easiest way to understand the statistical principles associated with each one. Figure 4-a shows there is a likelihood of a point equal to 0.135% to happen when it is out of the interval. This is an example of the rule 1 violation. Figure 4-b displays an example where the second rule is violated. In this case, the probability for one point more than 2*s* from the center line is calculated adding the probability equal to 2.14% with 0.135%, which is equal to a probability of 2.28%. The probability for two points more than 1*s* from the center line is the square of 2.28% which is equal to 0.0518%. The probability for the third point is calculated subtracting 2.28% from 100% = 97.72%. The probability for two out of three is determined according to $2.28^2\% \cdot 97.72\% \cdot 3 = 0.152\%$. Figure 4-c illustrates the case where rule 3 is violated. The probability for one point higher than 1*s* from the center line is the sum of 13.60%, 2.14%, and 0.135%, which is equal to 15.88%. The probability for four points to be more than 1*s* from the center line is $15.88^4\% = 0.0635\%$. The likelihood for the fifth point is calculated summing 2 · 34.13%, 13.60%, 2.14%, and 0.135%, which is equal to 84.14% or subtracting 15.88% from 100%. The probability of the four out of five is the calculated multiplying $15.88^4\%$, 84.12%, and five; the probability is equal to 0.267%. The example of rule 4 violation is seen in Figure 4-d The probability for one point is equal to the sum of 34.13%, 13.60%, 2.14%, and 0.135% = 50%. The probability for two points is the square of 50% = 25%. The sample square criteria sequence is applied to the other points, where the eighth point is equal to $50^8\% = 0.39\%$.

Alternatively, could be applied for the *R*-chart a simpler set of two rules:
Rule 1. One or more points beyond the UCL_R, and;
Rule 2. Two-thirds or more of the values of the ranges are below the average range $\overline{R}$.

Also, for the x or $\bar{x}$-chart could be used alternatively five rules:

Rule 1. One or more points beyond the control limits *UCL* or *LCL*;

Rule 2. Seven or more consecutive points increasing or decreasing: trend;

Rule 3. Eight or more consecutive points on one side of the average $\bar{x}$ or $\bar{\bar{x}}$

Rule 4. At least two out of three consecutive points beyond two-thirds of *UCL* or *LCL*, and;

Rule 5. At least four out of five consecutive points beyond one-third of *UCL* or *LCL* (entry 6.2.4 of [25]).

So, what set of rules should be used? The answer could not be universal since it depends on the stability of the process. Since it easy to apply any set of rules using a software such as Minitab®, it is suggestd the use of the "zone rules" for generally all the processes to produce blood components. The use of complementary rules could be a source of false alarms since the production of blood components is usually stable.

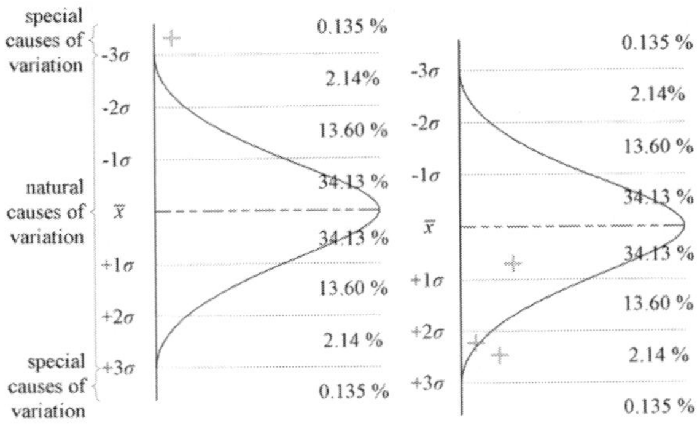

a. Rule 1 b. Rule 2

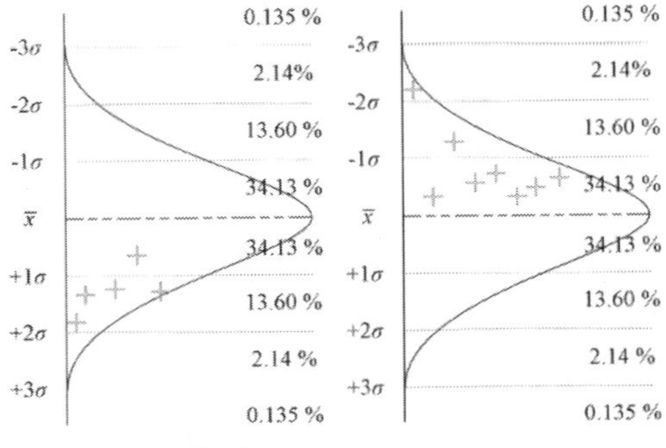

c. Rule 3 d. Rule 4

Figure 4. Cases of alarms for each of the decision "zone rules."

6.3. Control Charts for Attributes

6.3.1. Types of Control Charts

Control chart for attributes is used when it is no practicable to measure a certain characteristic, e.g., when the data distribution is not normal. The input is a count of the characteristic instead a measurement. For example, the number of red blood components non-conforming to hematocrit instead to measure the average and range. The classification of attribute results is according to the state of conformity, i.e., no/yes, non-conforming/conforming. Mostly, p-charts and c-charts are applied. p-charts consider the ratio of the attribute in a sampling. For example, if a sampling has $n = 4$ and one sample has a non-conforming hematocrit result, the ratio is 0.25 or 25%. c-charts consider the count of defective samples. For example, using the same case, the count is equal to one. These charts are complementary.

6.3.2. p-Charts with Fixed Rational Subgroup

The center line is equal to the average of the number of process fraction nonconforming $\overline{p}$. The mathematical model is correspondent to the Equation (3) (entry 7.2 of [25]):

$$\overline{p} = \frac{\sum_{i=1}^{m} D_i}{mn} = \frac{\sum_{i=1}^{m} \hat{p}_i}{m} \tag{26}$$

where p_i is the ratio of nonconforming samples i, $i = 1,\ldots,m$, m is the number of rational subgroups, and n is sample size per rational subgroup. The sample size is selected to assure an adequate sensitivity to detect non-conforming products. Therefore, it is assumed that m should be no less than 20.

The control limits, the upper control limit $UCL_{\overline{p}}$ and the lower control limit $LCL_{\overline{p}}$, are computed using the following models:

$$UCL_{\overline{p}} = \overline{p} + 3\sqrt{\frac{\overline{p}(1-\overline{p})}{n}} \tag{27}$$

$$LCL_{\overline{p}} = \overline{p} - 3\sqrt{\frac{\overline{p}(1-\overline{p})}{n}} \tag{28}$$

where $\overline{p}$ is the average of the ratio of nonconforming samples, and n is the number of samples per the rational subgroup.

For example, let consider the number of leucocytes in 30 lots with a fixed quantity of samples per sampling of *red cells, leucocyte depleted in additive solution* components ($m = 25$). It is assumed that leucocytes have a logarithmic distribution. This rational subgroup is from a blood establishment where it is produced a daily lot where the sampling is according to the significantly different number of blood components produced. Figure 5 shows the p-chart, and the data is displayed in Table 8. Equation (26) determines the center line, and Equations (27) and (28) and the control limits of p-chart charts as follows:

$$\overline{p} = \frac{\sum_{i=1}^{30} D_i}{25(30)} = \frac{2}{750} = 0.00267\ ,$$

$$UCL_{\overline{p}} = 0.00267 + 3\sqrt{\frac{0.00267(1-0.00267)}{25}} = 0.03361\ ,$$

and; $LCL_{\overline{p}} = 0$ (note: since $LCL_{\overline{p}} < 0$ it is assumed to be equal to zero)

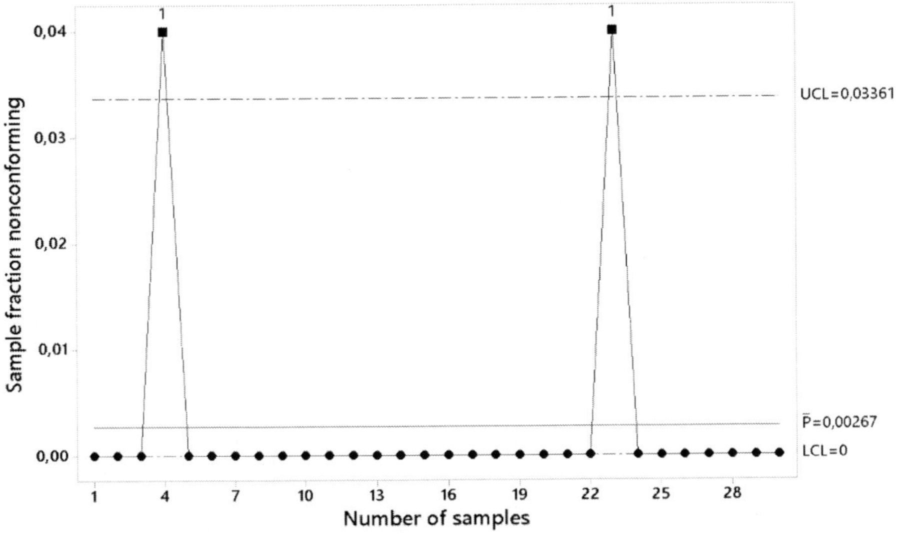

Figure 5. p-charts for the control of the leucocytes count of in a series of rational subgroups with a fixed number of samples.

Table 8. Variable sampling of *red cells, leucocyte depleted in additive solution* components

No.	D_i	$\hat{p}_i$	No.	D_i	$\hat{p}_i$	No.	D_i	$\hat{p}_i$
1	0	0	11	0	0	21	0	0
2	0	0	12	0	0	22	0	0
3	0	0	13	0	0	23	1	0.04
4	1	0.04	14	0	0	24	0	0
5	0	0	15	0	0	25	0	0
6	0	0	16	0	0	26	0	0
7	0	0	17	0	0	27	0	0
8	0	0	18	0	0	28	0	0
9	0	0	19	0	0	29	0	0
10	0	0	20	0	0	30	0	0
			$\sum D_i = 2$			$\bar{p} = 0.00267$		

6.3.3. np-Charts Fixed Rational Subgroup

The center line is equal to the average of the number of the defectives in sampling $\bar{p}$. The model derives from the Equation 26, as follows (entry 7.2 of [25]):

$$n\bar{p} = \bar{p}(n) \tag{29}$$

where $\bar{p}$ is the average of the number of process fraction nonconforming, and n is the number of samples of the rational subgroup.

The control limits, the upper control limit $UCL_{\overline{np}}$, and the lower control limit $LCL_{\overline{np}}$, are calculated using the following models:

$$UCL_{n\bar{p}} = n\bar{p} + 3\sqrt{n\bar{p}(1-\bar{p})} \tag{30}$$

$$LCL_{n\bar{p}} = n\bar{p} - 3\sqrt{n\bar{p}(1-\bar{p})} \tag{31}$$

where $\bar{p}$ is the average of the ratio of nonconforming samples, and n is the number of samples of the rational subgroup.

The previous example used to the *np*-charts is shown in Figure 6. Equation (29) determines the center line, and Equations (30) and (31) and the control limits of *np*-chart charts as follows:

$n\bar{p} = 0.002667(25) = 0.067$, $UCL_{n\bar{p}} = 0.066667 + 3\sqrt{0.066667(1-0.002667)} = 0.840$, and; $LCL_{n\bar{p}} = 0$ (note: since $LCL_{n\bar{p}} < 0$ it is assumed to be equal to zero)

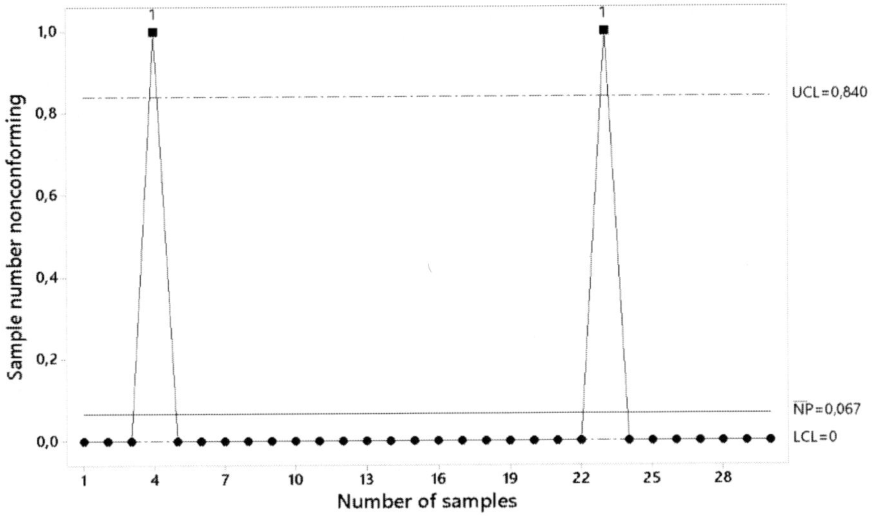

Figure 6. *np*-charts for the control of the leucocytes count of in a series of rational subgroups with a fixed number of samples.

6.3.4. Interpreting Control Charts

Dumont et al. published a paper regarding the control of leukocytes in a type of blood components [26]. It is argued the use of *n*, confidence interval, and the α-error define the number of acceptable rejections using non-parametric results of laboratory tests. This methodology is related to the probability of rejection zone and the probability of error detection. These topics are not discussed in this Chapter. In this approach, the lot must have no less than 25 samples. For example, if it the lot is equal to 25 samples, it is selected α-error equal to 10% and a confidence level equal to 90% (see Table 9). If the user prefers to decrease the α-error or to increase the confidence interval, the number of the sample must be increased. This not a problematic since existing retrospective data informing that a certain method of production is systematically stable. Another case, if the α-error is equal to 5% and the confidence level is equal to 95%, the minimum sample size is 100. If there is more than one rejection, it is assumed that a special cause is happening.

Table 9. Acceptable number of rejections in data not parametrically distributed considering the number of samples, confidence interval (CI), and the α-error

	α-error = 1%			α-error = 5%			α-error = 10%		
n	CI = 90%	CI = 95%	CI = 99%	CI = 90%	CI = 95%	CI = 99%	CI= 90%	CI = 95%	CI = 99%
25	-	-	-	-	-	-	0	-	-
50	-	-	-	0	-	-	≤2	≤1	0
100	-	-	-	≤2	≤1	0	≤6	≤5	≤3
150	-	-	-	≤4	≤3	≤2	≤10	≤9	≤7
200	-	-	-	≤6	≤4	≤3	≤14	≤13	≤10
300	0	0	-	≤10	≤8	≤6	≤23	≤21	≤18
400	≤1	0	-	≤14	≤12	≤10	≤32	≤30	≤26
500	≤2	≤1	0	≤18	≤17	≤13	≤41	≤39	≤35
750	≤3	≤2	≤1	≤29	≤27	≤23	≤64	≤61	≤56
1000	≤5	≤4	≤3	≤41	≤38	≤34	≤87	≤84	≤78

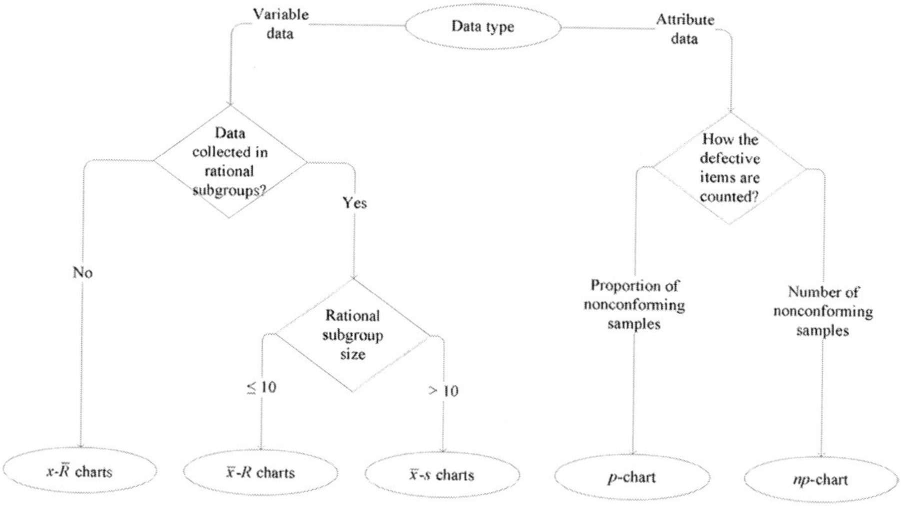

Figure 7. Flowchart to select the type of chart in the control of the blood components production.

6.3.5. Selection of a Chart

The quality control manager considers $\overline{x}$-R variables charts if a new process of production starts or if a new blood component starts to be manufactured. These charts are also applied when an old process shows long-term problems. They are also useful when for diagnostic purposes, when a test is destructive, when very tight specifications are used, or when are deciding about adjustments to the process. x-$\overline{R}$ charts are advantageous when it is difficult to group samples, when full testing is required or when the data rate is too slow.

The attributes charts are selected when it is intended to reduce the process fallout. Its role is also valuable to the evaluation of multiple step process. Perceptibly, when variables are unmeasurable, the attribute charts are an alternative. They could also have an important role when is performed a historical synopsis of the process. Figure 7 displays a diagram to select the chart following what is discussed in this Chapter.

7. PROCESS CAPABILITY

7.1. Process Capability Indexes

The process capability indexes classify the ability of an in-control process to satisfy the goals. They should be only applied to stable/controlled processes. The indexes inform how often the process fits into the specifications. It is determined originally using $\hat{C}_p$ which is determined by the model:

$$\hat{C}_p = \frac{USL - LSL}{6\hat{\sigma}} \tag{32}$$

where USL is the specified upper limit, LSL is the specified lower limit and $\hat{\sigma}$ is the estimated variability of the process (within limits standard deviation). Since the standard deviation is biased, $\hat{\sigma}$ is more accurately determined if is the outcome of the division of the $\overline{R}$ for each rational subgroup by d_2 which is the statistical coefficient of correlation selected according to rational subgroups from Table 4 (for sigma estimate). If it is used $\overline{x} - s$ chart, the division is similar, where $\overline{R}$ is replaced by s and d_2 by C_4 (see Table 4 for sigma estimate). The $\hat{C}_p$ model is adapted from the theoretical C_p since the process sigma σ is practically unmeasurable and is replaced by an estimate of standard deviation.

C_p classifies how the distribution of the results fits within the specification limits. This index represents the relation of the range of the specification limits with the range of the process. There is no information if the process is within specification. The value is always positive. The $\hat{C}_p$ index could be interpreted as:

If $\hat{C}_p = 1$, indicates that the process variation just meets specifications, i.e., the process to produce a certain blood component is minimally capable;

If $\hat{C}_p < 1$, indicates that the process variation is outside the specification range, i.e., the process is not capable to produce a certain blood component within specification and it needs to be improved, and;

If $\hat{C}_p > 1$, indicates that process variation is tighter than specifications and it surpasses minimal capability, i.e., the process is capable and the current practices are to maintain.

Let consider the example of the average and range charts (see 6.2.2), where the specification limit is [0.5,0.7]. In this case, the calculus is as follows:

$$\hat{C}_p = \frac{0.7-0.5}{6\left(\frac{0.02733}{1.693}\right)} = 2.07$$

Since $\hat{C}_p > 1$, this process is at the best ranking.

$\hat{C}_{pk}$ is another model to determine the capability index. It represents how centered is the data between the specification limits. To determine $\hat{C}_{pk}$ when is used a specification interval with a single limit, it is determined the $\hat{C}_{pk,upper}$ to the upper specification limit or the $\hat{C}_{pk,lower}$ to the lower specification limit using the models:

$$\hat{C}_{pk,upper} = \frac{USL-\hat{\mu}}{3\hat{\sigma}} \tag{33}$$

$$\hat{C}_{pk,lower} = \frac{\hat{\mu}-LSL}{3\hat{\sigma}} \tag{34}$$

where $\hat{\mu}$ is the production process average, and $\hat{\sigma}$ is the estimated variability of the process (within standard deviation). $\hat{C}_{pk}$ is equal to the lower index. To determine $\hat{C}_{pk}$ when is used a specification interval with double limits, first, it is determined the $\hat{C}_{pk,upper}$ and $\hat{C}_{pk,lower}$. Afterward, it is selected the minimum index:

$$\hat{C}_{pk} = \min\left[\hat{C}_{pk,upper}, \hat{C}_{pk,lower}\right] \tag{35}$$

The C_{pk} index could be interpreted as:

If $\hat{C}_{pk} < 1$, indicates that the process is inadequate, i.e., the process is not capable of producing reliable blood components;

If $1 \leq \hat{C}_{pk} < 1.33$, indicates that the process is capable, but a rigorous quality control is required, i.e., the process producing a certain blood component is minimally capable;

If $1.33 \leq \hat{C}_{pk} < 1.5$, indicates that the process is satisfactory, indicating that no severe quality control is required;

If $1.5 \leq \hat{C}_{pk} < 2$, indicates that the process is excellent, no stringent quality control is required;

If $\hat{C}_{pk} \geq 2$, indicates that the process is super, minimal quality control is required.

For example, considering the previous case (see 6.2.2):

$$\hat{C}_{pk} = \min\left[\frac{0.7 - 0.60022}{3\left(\frac{0.02733}{1.693}\right)}, \frac{0.60022 - 0.5}{3\left(\frac{0.02733}{1.693}\right)}\right] = 2.06$$

This could be interpreted as the index with the average closest to the specification limit. The C_{pk} index is the relation of the difference between the range of the specification limit (or vice-versa) and the average of the process to the range of the process. If the value is below one, there are values outside specification. If the value is exactly equal to zero, half of the values are out of the specification.

Regularly, the $\hat{C}_{pk}$ is chosen over $\hat{C}_p$ since it has a recognized limitation: to assume that the process variability is centered on the specification extension, which is not true in all the cases. $\hat{C}_{pk}$ is statistically reliable in this condition. When a process is centered, $\hat{C}_p$ is equal to $\hat{C}_{pk}$. Both indexes should never be estimated from a small number of samples since the results are not realistic due to the sampling is not statistically representative of the production. If C_p index is higher than C_{pk}, the process is off-center [27].

The process performance indexes, P_p, and P_{pk}, classify how well the data fits within the specification limits, and classify how centered the data is between the specification limits. They are intended to be used when the total production is known the laboratory is testing the performance of a production method. The mathematical models differs in the use of standard deviation instead a ratio of $\bar{R}/d_2$ or s/C_4

P_p is computed using a model similar to C_p:

$$\hat{P}_p = \frac{USL - LSL}{6s} \tag{36}$$

where USL is the specified upper limit, LSL is the specified lower limit, and s is the standard deviation of the overall results (overall standard deviation). Such as $\hat{C}_p$, $\hat{P}_p$ is not useful to identify in the process out-of-specifications. P_p and C_p results differ due to the within rational subgroup standard deviation to be lower than the $\bar{R}/d_2$. Both have the same limitation regarding the centralization, which is considered by none. They could be uniquely determined when USL and LSL limits exist, for what they cannot be applied to some of the parameters utilized to control the production of blood components.

Let use the case from 6.2.2:

$$\hat{P}_p = \frac{0.7 - 0.5}{6(0.01572)} = 2.12$$

P_{pk} calculus is identical to the C_{pk}, differing also in the use of the s instead $\hat{\sigma}$. It is determined using the model:

$$\hat{P}_{pk,upper} = \frac{USL - \bar{x}}{3s} \tag{37}$$

$$\hat{P}_{pk,lower} = \frac{\overline{x} - LSL}{3s} \tag{38}$$

where $\overline{x}$ is the production process average. $\hat{P}_{pk}$ is equal to the lower index. To determine $\hat{P}_{pk}$ when is used a specification interval with double limits, first, it is determined the $\hat{P}_{pk,upper}$ and $\hat{P}_{pk,lower}$. Afterward, it is selected the minimum index, $\hat{P}_{pk} = \min\left[\hat{P}_{pk,upper}, \hat{P}_{pk,lower}\right]$.

For example,

$$\hat{P}_{pk} = \min\left[\frac{0.7-0.60022}{3(0.01572)}, \frac{0.60022-0.5}{3(0.01572)}\right] = 2.12$$

In the $\hat{P}_p$ and $\hat{P}_{pk}$ examples, the indexes are not considerably different from $\hat{C}_p$ and $\hat{C}_{pk}$.

The difference between C_p and P_p and C_{pk} and P_{pk} is not significant if the distribution is normal and the process is in-control since the difference between the within standard deviation ($\overline{R}/d_2$) and overall standard deviation (s) is minor. However, in the cases with unnatural sources of variation, the C_{pk} index is higher than the P_{pk}. Despite the process performance indexes are recommended by the Automotive Industry Action Group (AIAG) and the American Society for Quality Control, they are not consensual. Some authors do not recommend its use, classifying the approach as "statistical terrorism" [27] and arguing "they are a waste of engineering and management effort - they tell you nothing" (entry 8.3.5 of [25]). This Chapter suggests its use along with C_p and C_{pk}. C_p and C_{pk} indexes should be close in the P_p and P_{pk} result. If C_p and C_{pk} are significantly higher than P_p or P_{pk} (minimum one-third higher), the process could not be stable enough to compute the capability indexes. In this case, the evaluation of the stability of process is done principally using charts instead capability indexes, using a rigorous quality control strategy.

Table 10 shows a set of examples where the analysis of P_{pk} is valuable to better understand the capability of the process. Figures 10-a to d shows a set of cases where the average in around the center line. Figure 10-a illustrates a case where the process is super with C_{pk} and P_{pk} indexes higher than two. Figure 10-b displays an example where the process is capable with C_{pk} and P_{pk} indexes between one and 1.33. Figure 10-c demonstrate the case of a non-capable process due to both lower indexes. Figure 10-d shows an example where according to the C_{pk} index the process is classified as super, but according to the P_{pk} the process is non-capable. The difference is due to the computing models of within standard deviation and overall standard deviation. The process must be carefully monitored using control charts and decision rules. Figure 10-e illustrates a case of shit from the center line with data with the low standard deviation (similar to the results of Figure 10-a standard deviation) with an insignificant difference between estimates. Finally, Figure 10-f illustrates the case where the within and overall standard deviation are close (identical to the estimates in Figure 10-b) and less than one. The capability is influenced in this example by a shift from the center line.

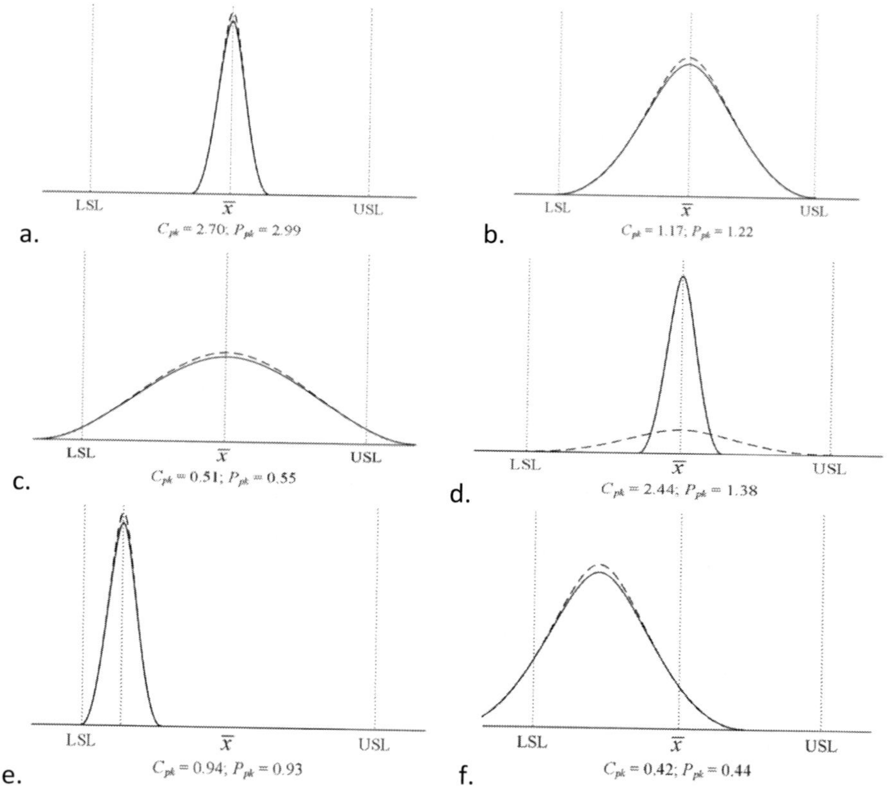

Figure 8. Flowchart to select the type of chart in the control of the blood components production.

7.2. Sigma Capability

Sigma stands for the number of the standard deviation of a certain process. A 3-sigma process has 2600 parts per million (ppm) defective, and it is acknowledged as the minimum capability index in production. A 6-sigma process has uniquely 3.4 ppm defective. Consequently, a 6-sigma process has a lower chance to manufacture out-of-specification products when compared to a 3-sigma process. Sigma could be computed, simply multiplying C_{pk} by three. The sigma levels are classified as follows:

6-sigma ($C_{pk} = 2$) as "world class quality";
5-sigma ($C_{pk} = 1.66$) as the goal related to quality improvement;
4-sigma ($C_{pk} = 1.33$) as the typical sigma level in industry, and;
3-sigma ($C_{pk} = 1$) as the minimum acceptable quality level.

Accordingly, typically required performance is around 4-sigma. As it can be seen, the classifications are close to the C_{pk} levels. Usually, the first goal in a sigma project is to change from a 4 to a 5-sigma performance, i.e., change the process performance from satisfactory to excellent. The blood components production has some parameters with a performance higher than 6-sigma, equivalent to "world class quality." However, some never achieve a high sigma level, principally due to the biological variation of the parameters tested. For further details about 6-sigma concept, please refer to [29].

CONCLUSION

Summarizing, this Chapter briefly discusses and demonstrate an SPC methodology as a critical tool to the control of blood components production. Part of the most significant models to the control of blood components quality are featured. Since it is required expertise in the fields of blood components production, statistics, and SPC, its successful implementation is a challenge for most blood establishments. Therefore, its application could effectively occur uniquely if supported and maintained by trained personnel. To start an application of an SPC methodology out of this condition is understood as a bad practice assuring a weak control of the process. The theory and examples presented are intended to assist the blood establishment laboratorian in understanding the major concepts based on empirical data studies. The user could easily apply the approaches using an SPC dedicated software, or alternatively, using a spreadsheet software.

REFERENCES

[1] Commission Directive 2002/98/EC of the European Parliament and of the Council as regards setting standards of quality and safety for the collection, testing, processing, storage and distribution of human blood and blood components and amending Directive 2001/83/EC. Official Journal of the European Union L33/30-40.

[2] American Association of Blood Banks. Standards for blood banks and transfusion services. 30th ed. Bethesda (MD): American Association of Blood Banks, 2016.

[3] European Directorate for the Quality of Medicines and HealthCare. Guide to the preparation, use and quality assurance of blood components. 18th ed. Strasbourg: EDQM;2015.

[4] Pereira P, Westgard J, Encarnação P, Seghatchian J, Sousa G. Quality management in the European screening laboratories in blood establishments: a view on current approaches and trends. *Transfusion and Apheresis Science* 2015; 52(2) 245-251. DOI: 10.1016/j.transci. 2015.02.014.

[5] Pereira P, Westgard J, Encarnação P, Seghatchian J, de Sousa G. The role of uncertainty in results of screening immunoassays in blood establishments. *Transfusion and Apheresis Science* 2015; 52(2) 252-255. DOI: 10.1016/j.transci.2015.02.015kjl.

[6] Bureau International des Poids et Mesures. JCGM 200:2012 International vocabulary of metrology - Basic and general concepts and associated terms, 2008 version with minor corrections. 3rd ed. Sèvres: BIPM; 2012. Retrieved from http://www.bipm.org/utils/common/ documents/jcgm/JCGM_200_2012.pdf. Accessed: April 25, 2016.

[7] Statistical quality control handbook. 2nd ed. Western Electric Company, Inc.; 1958.

[8] Conti T. Systems thinking: the new frontier in quality management. Proceedings of the 53rd Congress of European Organization for Quality, May 12-14, 2009; Dubrovnik, Croatia. Retrieved from http://www.eoq. org/fileadmin/user_upload/Documents/Congress_proceedings/Croatia_ May_2009/Proceedings/Conti.pdf. Accessed: April 25, 2016.

[9] International Organization for Standardization. ISO 9000 Quality management systems - Fundamentals and vocabulary. 4th ed. Geneva: ISO; 2015.

[10] European Directorate for the Quality of Medicines and HealthCare. The collection, testing and use of blood and blood components in Europe. Strasbourg: EDQM;2012. Retrieved from https://www.edqm.eu/sites/default/files/the_collection_testing_and_use_of_blood_and_blood_components_in_europe_2012_report.pdf. Accessed: April 25, 2016.

[11] International Organization for Standardization. ISO 9001 Quality management systems - Requirements. 5th ed. Geneva: ISO; 2015.

[12] Saaty T. Decision making with the analytic hierarchy process. *International Journal of Services Sciences* 2008; 1(1) 83-98. DOI: 10.1504/IJSSCI.2008.017590.

[13] Pereira P. An analytical hierarchy process to decision making in human blood, cells, and tissue banks. In: Applications and theory of analytic hierarchy process. Rijeka: InTech; 2016.

[14] Fraser C. Biological variation: from principles to practice. Washington (DC): AACC Press 2001.

[15] Wheeler D. Two Definitions of Trouble. Manuscript no. 203 (Quality Digest). Knoxville (TN): Statistical Process Controls, Inc.;2009.

[16] Thompson S. Sampling. 3rd ed. New York (NY): John Wiley and Sons, Inc.; 2012.

[17] International Organization for Standardization. ISO 3951 Sampling procedures for inspection by variables - Part 1: Specification for single sampling plans indexed by acceptance quality limit (AQL) for lot-by-lot inspection for a single quality characteristic and a single AQL. 2nd ed. Geneva: ISO; 2013.

[18] D'Agostino, R. Transformation to normality of the null distribution of g1. *Biometrika* 1970; 57(3):679-681. DOI:10.1093/biomet/57.3.679.

[19] International Organization for Standardization. ISO 16269 Statistical interpretation of data - Part 4: Detection and treatment of outliers. Geneva: ISO; 2010.

[20] Grubbs, F. Procedures for detecting outlying observations in samples. *Technometrics* 1969,11(1):1-21.

[21] Rosner, B. Percentage points for a generalized ESD many-outlier procedure. *Technometrics* 1983,25(2):165-172.

[22] Tukey, J. Exploratory data analysis. Reading (MA): Addison-Wesley Publishing Company;1977.

[23] Quesenberry, C. An SPC approach to compensating a tool-wear process. *Journal of Quality Technology* 1988,20(4):220-229.
[24] MacGregor, J; Kourti, T. Statistical process control of multivariate processes. *Control Engineering Practice* 1995, 3(3):403-414.
[25] Montgomery, D. Introduction to statistical quality control. 7th ed. New York (NY): John Wiley and Sons, Inc.; 2012.
[26] Dumont, L; Dzik W; Rebulla, P; Brandwein, H. Practical guidelines for process validation and process control of white cell-reduced blood components: report of the Biomedical Excellence for Safer Transfusion (BEST) Working Party of the International Society of Blood Transfusion (ISBT). *Transfusion* 1996,36(1):11-20.
[27] Kotz, S; Lovelace, C. Process Capability Indices in Theory and Practice. London: Arnold; 1998.
[28] George, M. Lean 6-sigma: combining 6-sigma quality with Lean production speed. New York (NY): The McGraw-Hill Companies, Inc.; 2012. DOI: 10.1036/0071385215.

In: Blood Donations
Editor: Antoinette Luna

ISBN: 978-1-63485-457-3

Chapter 4

USE OF MODERN TEST THEORETICAL INSTRUMENTS (ITEM RESPONSE THEORY: IRT) AT FIRST TIME IN OBJECTIVE MEASUREMENT OF NURSES' TRANSFUSION-RELATED KNOWLEDGE – A HUNGARIAN SURVEY

Veronika Rajki [*] ***and Mária Csóka***
Department of Nursing, Faculty of Health Sciences,
Semmelweis University, Budapest, Hungary

ABSTRACT

The role of nurses in transfusion therapy continues to increase. A set of reliable measurement tools is required to assess various components of the professional knowledge including factual knowledge, skills and competence as outcomes of nursing education and training. Traditional questionnaires and test methods do not allow the measurement of these characteristics properly, as these tools typically provide overall scores without relevant insight into areas in which nurses perform well, and those where their knowledge and/or skills should be improved substantially. Our nationwide survey took place between November 19,

[*] Vas str. 17., Budapest, H-1088, Hungary Email: rajki.veronika@se-etk.hu.

2014 and February 20, 2015. Data were collected using paper-form and web-based anonymous, self-administered questionnaire. 657 nurses who were involved in transfusion therapy with changing regularity in adult in-patient wards took part in the survey. Data were processed using descriptive statistical methods. The knowledge and skills of 657 participants were assessed using a validated instrument consisting of a set of questions covering every aspects of transfusion therapy. The answers to these items were evaluated on a binary scale. Recorded answers of the participants were analyzed using hierarchical cluster analysis and item response theory tools such as the one-parametric Rasch model suitable for dichotomous data. Data analysis was performed with the SPSS program and the ltm module of the R statistical program. It was found that the transfusion therapy related knowledge of nurses was very incomplete (50.72%), and only about half of the nurses (52.3%) systematized the nursing functions correctly. The vast majority of the institutions had their own protocol, but responsible nurses assigned for transfusion care were present only in 23.9% of the wards. The paper presents the distribution of correct and incorrect answers to various questions about transfusion therapy along with the corresponding logit values and odds ratios, respectively. The characteristic curves of each item were determined on the basis of the number of correct answers that have been recorded. These curves highlight which questions were answered easily and which items were found harder to answer by the nurses who participated in the survey. In addition to the separate analysis of individual questions, a set of response patterns is also presented which shows how frequently the nurses responded correctly to different combinations (sub-sets) of questions. On the whole, nurses exhibited medium level performance in terms of knowledge and skills required for efficient and safe transfusion practice. The authors conclude that the identified problems can be resolved by improving professional responsibility of nurses, increasing supervision by nursing leaders and appropriate transfusiology training and regular retrainings. Objective and reliable measurement of the level of acquired knowledge is a key requirement in nursing education. This paper, which demonstrates the use of cluster analysis and item response theory for the assessment of transfusion-related knowledge of nurses, focuses on this issue for the first time in nursing research. The results of this survey have revealed substantial limitations and deficiencies both in knowledge and skills of nurses which need to be addressed by training in order to improve the efficiency and safety of transfusion therapy.

Keywords: nursing competency, transfusion-related knowledge, blood safety, patient safety, modern test theory, knowledge measurement, cluster analysis, Rasch model

INTRODUCTION

In this day and age, safe blood transfusions (haemovigilance, blood safety) are an immediate, global, and extremely important issue in the field of health care system. France has the pioneering work on haemovigilance, it started in France in 1994. From the beginning the monitoring systems were used by Blood Transfusion Committees and a national haemovigilance system was established. In 1995 the European Council published a resolution with the aim of improving public confidence in safe blood supply. Nowadays the best known haemovigilance systems in various countries are the following ones: United Kingdom (Serious Hazards of Transfusion [SHOT]), Canada (Transfusion Transmitted Injuries Surveillance System [TTISS]), Netherlands (Transfusion Reactions in Patients [TRIP]). [10, 23] "Haemovigilance is required to identify and prevent occurrence or recurrence of transfusion related unwanted events, to increase the safety, efficacy and efficiency of blood transfusion, covering all activities of the transfusion chain from donor to recipient." [23] As with other areas within the health care system, the field of blood transfusion therapy, likewise, encounters unexpected situations within which dangers may undermine patient safety and security, and destabilize the entire system. Therefore required to report and publish the variety of (serious) adverse events, for example, blood transfusion errors. The no-blame cultural approach is/would be also very important in health care system. [24] Blood quality is directly related to the safety of therapy, product safety, as well as the preparative and clinical transfusiology' entire process. The principle actors involved with transfusion therapy, namely the nurses, are professionally, legally and ethically responsible for their own conduct. Foreign professional literature mutually affirms that the increasingly important role of nurses involved in tranfusion therapy is not only growing but that the nurses' role is fundamental to the continued maintenance of blood quality and successful therapy. [7, 9, 16] Due to an international guidance which was published by the Nursing and Midwifery Council in 2007, a key requirement is that all staff involved in blood transfusion undergo formal competency assessment on a three-yearly basis. [16] Within the current national context, nurses' roles and responsibilities should be increased so as to partake and become more involved in the transfusion process. [2, 16] In as such, the nurses' professional role would include a strong corresponding skill set, willingness to perform, and precise work.

In addition to this, it is important that nurses are not only aware of their own competencies but comply with their competency requirements. The understanding and definition of the competencies are unquestionably a key function of nursing standards.

Blood transfusion safety is a relevant and an extremely important theme in health care systems nowadays. Unfortunately, transfusion-related mistakes, mistransfusion events reported can happen and these are reported to the responsible organizations/professional bodies. For example, the Serious Hazards of Transfusion (SHOT) scheme is a UK-wide, independent, professionally led haemovigilance system focused on learning from adverse events. “SHOT was established in 1996 as a confidential reporting system for significant transfusion-related events, building an evidence base to support blood safety policy decisions, clinical guidelines, clinician education, and improvements in transfusion practice. Recommendations are formulated by an independent steering group drawn from medical royal colleges and professional bodies” [21].

SHOT is a professional, anonymised reporting system, which collects data about serious issues concerning the transfusion of blood components in order to:

- Aid the production of national clinical and laboratory guidelines for the use of blood
- educate users in transfusion hazards and their prevention
- improve standards of hospital transfusion practice
- inform policy in transfusion services and aid the production of clinical guidelines on the use of blood components” [19].

The reported data was alarming: upon the inception of SHOT, event reporting rates increased from 22 percent in 1996 to 98.4 percent in 2011. Within this ’anonymous’ context, event reporting rose from 4.8 events per 10,000 components in 2007 to 11.6 events per 10,000 components in 2011. Within this period, it is estimated that over 3,000 incorrect blood transfused cases had occurred and had been reported. This includes, but is not limited to: situations in which patients were transfused with inappropriate blood components; blood which was intended for another patient. These situations not only involved several miscalculations, but were preventable.

Acute transfusion reactions (ATR) represent the largest category of pathological and unforeseen events and was the leading cause of major morbidity in 2011 [18].

To promote and protect the interests and wellbeing of the patient, the Nursing and Midwifery Council (NMC) advise that the administration of medications "is not solely a mechanistic task to be performed in strict compliance with the written prescription of a medical practitioner (can now also be an independent and supplementary prescriber). It requires thought and the exercise of professional judgement" [16].

The role of the nurse in transfusion processes becomes clearer through their education while they become well-educated professionals/practitioners during this process. Nurses can demonstrate their skill and competency in this field, but they will need to undertake specific training, which can be provided either by the hospital, a trust or an external organization. The four UK health departments (2002) and SHOT (2004) recommended that every trust should employ a hospital transfusion practitioner, such as a specialist nurse or biomedical scientist. Hospital transfusion practitioners, in collaboration with lead consultants in blood transfusion and local blood bank managers support clinical teams in the safe and effective use of blood.

Transfusion practitioners also actively promote good transfusion practice by:

- "endorsing national guidelines and evidence-based practice
- facilitating transfusion audit and feedback (continuous improvement)
- facilitating incident reporting and follow up on any errors or near misses
- encouraging education/training and increasing clinical competency
- participating in the implementation of new technologies that enhance patient safety" [7, 9].

The National Transfusion Practitioner Survey of England and North Wales (2010) recommended that "a multifaceted approach is required to realize further improvements in patient safety and reduction in risk with respect to transfusion issues" [18].

The use of RFID (Radio Frequency IDentification) technology can also improve safety, quality and productivity in transfusion medicine. This has been explored at several institutions. *Figure 1* shows an example of an RFID-enabled process—transfusion [4].

Haemovigilance, according to the 2008 Hungarian Transfusion Regulations comprises a follow-up, and an all-encompassing system involving the entire transfusion process starting from blood collection to blood products production to patient (vein to vein) transfusion. This includes (monitoring for) seriously harmful or unexpected (adverse) events and serious complications concerning both the recipient and the donor, as well as the epidemiological monitoring of donors [17].

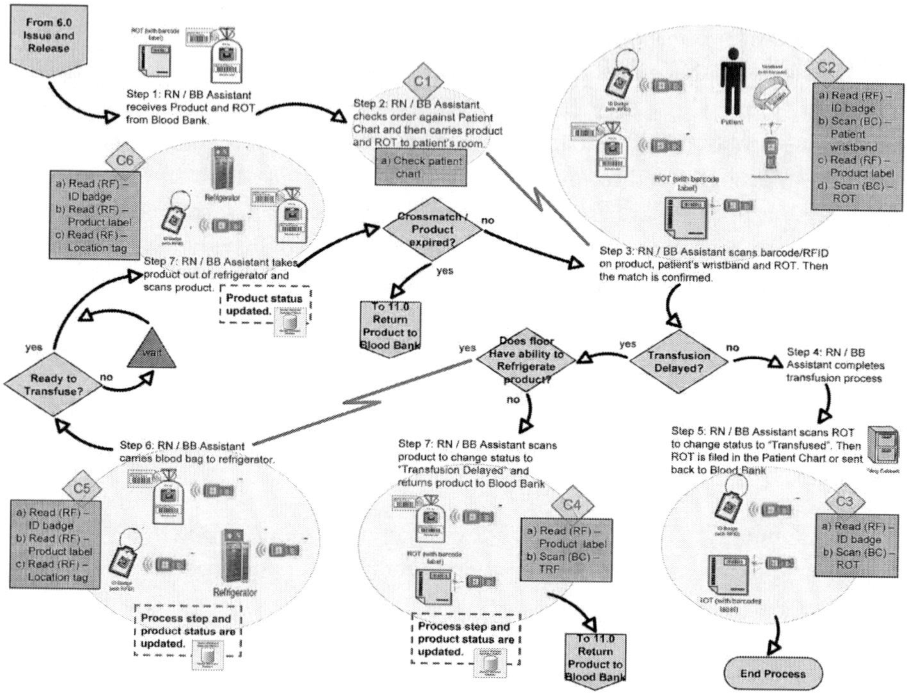

Figure 1. An example of an RFID-enabled process—transfusion [4].

In Spain, there has been a progressive increase in mistransfusion and incorrect blood component transfusion (ICBT) events reported to a local Regional Haemovigilance Division in recent years. Colleagues initiated a transfusion practice nursing survey to study the causes of the increasing mistransfusion rate. Mistransfusion rates between 2007 and 2009 were obtained from the Balearic Island Haemovigilance Division (BIHVD), one of the 17 regional HV divisions in the Spanish Haemovigilance network. Annually, approximately 47,000 transfusions are carried out by 614 nurses in this region. Data collection involved anonymous voluntary questionnaires with questions addressing socio-professional factors, transfusion training and education, together with transfusion practice questions both related and unrelated to guidelines and nurses' attitudes. They used multiple regression analysis to investigate which mistransfusion prediction factors were most accurate. The survey response rate was 363 out of 614 (59.12%). Realized deficits in nurses' education and training and low transfusion frequency had a strong negative impact on the incidence of transfusion errors ($r = \_0.70$; $p = 0.01$). This is supported by evidence that the performance of well-trained nurses who transfused either daily or weekly and strictly followed transfusion guidelines was associated with a lower mistransfusion rate ($r = \_0.93$; $p < 0.01$). In that survey it can be found that incorrect blood component transfusion (IBCT) occurrence is associated with poor nurse training and education, frequency of transfusion and a low level of knowledge. This study illustrates the feasibility of using Haemovigilance resources to investigate the causes of mistransfusion [11].

We can read the following recommendations about better and safer transfusions in the Report for the Australian Council for Safety and Quality in Health Care:

"Future investment in enhancing the safety of transfusion must address clinical transfusion practice improvement, not just blood product quality. In 2005 the major risks from transfusion are associated with unsafe clinical transfusion practices and inappropriate blood product transfusion.

Healthcare professionals involved in everyday transfusion practice must receive more adequate education and training to support safe and appropriate transfusion.

Australia should adopt a national clinical governance model for the safety and quality of blood and blood product transfusion. This would see organizations that currently contribute to aspects of the safety and quality of transfusion practice integrated within a single governance framework that addresses all aspects of the transfusion 'safety chain.'

A National Better, Safer Transfusion (BeST) program should be established to promulgate transfusion practice standards, oversee monitoring of transfusion performance and lead a parsimonious core of transfusion practice improvement activities. A national BeST Advisory Committee should develop this program. This Committee should report, via the Jurisdictional Blood Committee, to Australian Health Ministers.

This National Better, Safer Transfusion (BeST) program should operate through the normal accountability and responsibility channels of acute healthcare. Program implementation should be through jurisdictions. Jurisdictional BeST Committees with clear linkages to Hospital Transfusion Committees should work together on identified national transfusion safety and quality priorities.

Haemovigilance activities should be part of this National Better, Safer Transfusion (BeST) program.

Hospital Transfusion Committees and Hospital Transfusion Teams will only deliver enhanced transfusion safety and appropriateness if adequately resourced. This resourcing must include access to appropriately trained Medical staff and where relevant a trained Transfusion Nurse (or equivalent).

The safety and appropriateness of hospital transfusion practice should be an explicit responsibility of Executive Managers of Health Services" [3].

One survey dealing with transfusion therapy from the patient's perspective, though relatively rare, sought to identify how well patients understand the role of blood transfusion in their treatment and whether it causes them discomfort. 21 patients, who had received blood transfusion in an Ohio hospital over a five-week period in 2009, participated in semi-structured interviews lasting 15 to 30 minutes. All the participants were medically stable adults. The researchers recorded and transcribed the interviews and performed thematic analysis. Four themes emerged: paternalism and decision making, patients' knowledge, blood safety and administration, and the nurse's role.

Some examples from the patients' responses, according to this article, include:

In relation to paternalism and decision making:

- "I took their word that (blood transfusion) was necessary."
- "There is no question; the doctor says you need it ... you need it."
- "I trusted that the doctors were doing what they were supposed to do, what needed to be done. I didn't question the fact of them having to do it or the whole process in general."
- "Two doctors conferenced and made the decision."

In relation to patients' knowledge:

- "They did give me a pamphlet about blood transfusions."
- From a patient whose friend read the brochure: "She read a few things out loud to me so I understood what it was."
- "They just came in and said, 'You're getting a blood transfusion.' Yeah, yeah, it was kinda fast."
- "I just had to write a consent, or sign a consent."
- "I think it was a talk with the nurse and a brochure. I think that was it."

- "I got a pamphlet here that they gave me to read... . No, I did not [read it], just didn't feel like it."

In relation to blood safety and administration:

- "I had a lot of worries because ... they could have the disease ... and that's what the [patient brochure] says about risks, and I was worried about it."
- "After all the things you hear ... I didn't express the worry, but ... I think about it a little bit."
- "I appreciate the checklist, the comparing to my name tag, having two people do that. That was reassuring, to make sure I was getting the correct blood. It just relaxed me. I wasn't nervous about it beforehand, but it certainly added to the experience in a positive way."
- "In exactly 15 minutes that girl was back in here and checking everything she was supposed to."

In relation to the nurse's role:

- "I remember (the nurse) telling me about the [itchiness] and things like that."
- When the patient was asked who told her she needed a transfusion: "After having lab work done I was shopping and walking around for five hours. I got a call from the doctor's office, and it was the nurse. She told me to report to the hospital ED right away to be evaluated. My hemoglobin was 5.2. It was the nurse on the floor who said I need a transfusion."
- When the patient was asked about the blood administration process: "(The nurse) just hooked it up to my IV and it went so smooth. I had never been given blood before, and all the things you hear made me panic. I didn't express the worry, but she did it so good it was no big deal."
- "I asked if I really needed two bags. The nurse said to do the first one and to see how I feel. The nurse asked me if it was as bad as I thought it would be, and it wasn't. So she asked if I would like the second unit and I said sure, let's do it!"

Though a small convenience sample study, it had reported important conclusions. Results suggest that clinicians may be missing opportunities to improve patients' knowledge of, and comfort with, blood transfusions and that they can better meet patients' needs before, during, and after the procedure. This survey has highlighted weaknesses in practice. The researchers found that their participants said that nurses, more than other clinicians, advised patients on transfusions [22].

The goal of another study was to assess transfusion service staff attitudes about issues pertaining to event reporting and patient safety culture in the transfusion services. 945 transfusion service staff from 43 hospital transfusion services in the United States and 10 in Canada were involved in the survey. The overall response rate was 73 percent (693 responses). The study addresses issues such as: patient harm being reported (91%), mistakes not corrected that could cause harm (79%), less than one-third of respondents report deviations from procedures with no apparent potential for harm (31%), and mistakes that staff catch and correct on their own (27%). Staff indicated that the main reasons mistakes happen are interruptions (51%) and staff in other departments not knowing or understanding proper procedures (49%). Most of the staff were positive about their supervisor's safety actions and believed that their transfusion service tries to identify causes of mistakes. Only 31 % agreed that nursing staff would work with the transfusion service to reduce mistakes. This study provides useful information about how staff view event reporting and safety-related issues and identifies strengths and areas for improvement. [20]

The authors offered a closer look at transfusion reactions of nurses in the article. The appropriate professional reasons (for transfusion reactions) were the following: understanding the different types of transfusion reactions helps the nurse to relieve symptoms while addressing the cause of the reaction. This is very important because, in relation to any type of reaction, early recognition and prompt intervention are crucial [2].

We can read in an article from 2011 that modern transfusion therapy is not about us staff it is about the patient. This statement was mentioned as an indication of a very important international trend in transfusion therapy. In their opinion, another important trend in this regard is that more and more specialists concern themselves with patients who refuse blood transfusion [15].

The Blood Matters project started in April 2002. It commenced with the formation of a consortium composed of the then Victorian Department of Human Services, Peter MacCallum Cancer Institute, The Royal Melbourne Hospital and The Australian Red Cross Blood (the Blood Service). As their task, they developed and tested tools and processes to improve transfusion practice in hospitals. Also, the transfusion nurse's role was established in hospitals as part of the Blood Matters project. To support those in the role, The Blood Matters Consortium project developed a postgraduate certificate in transfusion practice.

The Postgraduate Certificate in Transfusion Practice is an online course administered by The University of Melbourne School of Nursing, and is coordinated by the Melbourne Consulting and Custom Programs. It consists of four subjects:

Semester one

- Fundamentals in Transfusion Practice
- Quality within Transfusion Practice

Semester two

- Advanced Concepts in Transfusion Practice
- Transfusion Specialty Practice (Clinical Practice Portfolio) [1]

As it can be found in the professional literature, a greater degree of involvement of nurses in transfusion therapy is suggested. However, this can be done only with serious professional skills and precise work by nurses.

The healthcare system's expectations do not focus so much on the memorized or written reproduction of knowledge, but rather on the practical knowledge required to address various types of situations, problems and solutions regarding individual patient cases and situations. [6] The results of training distinct skills – knowledge, practical skills and competencies – are determined by corresponding measurement instruments of those knowledge or proficiency skills [5].

Although traditional questionnaires and tests provided professionals with a means by which to measure the skill and knowledge sets and levels, by no means do these reflect or provide a clear picture of the 'real' or practical knowledge and skills needed. For this reason, for the successful teaching of these skills, as well as to know how effective the teaching was, a reliable instrument is required and is possible. [13] Current situations require distinct skills and knowledge sets as an objective, and likewise, reliable measurement (testing)instruments are necessary and possible. The Item Response Theory (IRT) provides a possible solution by addressing and measuring the individual skill competencies required in modern nursing scenarios [8, 12, 13, 14, 25].

Using a multi-level research approach– our aim was to focus on the measurement of blood donation and transfusion therapy practical errors which occur due to lack of knowledge. The reason for this aim is to outline those ways in which to improve the training of nurses by focusing on the errors and misunderstanding that take place in daily practice.

Based on the reasons stated earlier, two studies were conducted. We first explored four distinct professional groups (Adult nursing care-, Surgical care-, Emergency care-, Midwifery care professional group) in Hungary in 2012. The first study related to nurses ($N_{vo} = 312$) knowledge of blood donations as well as their attitudes and habits (preparative transfusiology survey). The second study (in 2014/2015) focused on the measurement of transfusion therapy nurses' knowledge, competencies ($N_{to} = 657$). These nurses work in adult transfusion therapy related (inpatient) institutes. The tests were focused on nurses' knowledge, job description, and local methods (clinical transfusiology survey). We created and validated a distinct measurement instrument for the latter study (clinical) prior to the national study conducted a few months earlier.

The data gathered in this cross-sectional study involved mathematical statistics and different descriptive methods and was presented in cluster analysis and multidimensional scaling tables in our second survey. We found that the use of these latter methods has not yet been used neither in national nor international literature. For these reasons, we anticipate that the results of this unique study adds to the research field in Hungary. In this chapter we introduce the results of our second survey.

AIMS OF THE SURVEY

In the field of clinical transfusion, it was our aim to measure nurses' transfusion therapy knowledge and practical skills through a survey. Our additional goal in the field of transfusion therapy, was to address and measure nurses' own competencies on a national level. Through comparison and contrast analysis, we aim to uncover the extent to which professionals comply with the existing specifications and requirements outlined in the Transfusion Regulations (2008).

In addition, the national survey was conducted so as to find out whether and to what extent the teaching goals correspond to actual nursing transfusion practice. We sought to exceed the classical test limitations and analyze in detail the nurses' professional transfusion skills. The objectives of instructors was to promote nurses' careers and success in the workplace, however, the results provided by traditional questionnaires are questionable in terms of representation of those skills. Our further goal, thus, was to create a new validated measurement instrument so as to objectively measure nurses' knowledge and skill base.

MATERIAL AND METHODS

The second survey used descriptive statistics, observation, questionnaires and interview approaches. The self-administered questionnaire was tested according to mathematical and statistical methods so as to establish reliability, validity, variation and standard deviation (SD), Cronbach alpha calculation and Pearson correlation determination coefficients. Questionnaire testing and re-testing was between July and August, 2014 ($n_j = 29$ and $n_a = 27$).

Between November 19, 2014 and February 20, 2015, we conducted a representative national study using our own questionnaire. Data collection (paper and anonymous web data) of self-administered questionnaires was conducted within standardized conditions using stratified sampling methods. The test samples or participants ($N_{to} = 657$) were nurses who worked with adult inpatient transfusion recipients receiving various and regular transfusion therapy. Descriptive statistics were first applied to the cross-sectional study data followed by mathematical statistics. In addition, the mathematical statistics were analyzed according to IBM SPSS (20. version) and the Microsoft Office 2013 program using cluster analysis and multidimensional scaling.

The objective measurement of nurses' skill sets were therefore measured by a validated measurement instrument (our questionnaire). According to regular tests, we could compare only raw data, but this would not provide an accurate picture of nurses' true knowledge and skill levels. We tried to eliminated the limitations of classical test by not addressing overall performance but by analyzing and focusing in detail (itemizing) their individual performance. The various aspects of transfusion practice were covered in a quiz that used binary (good/bad) scaling. The retrieved data was analyzed according to hierarchical cluster analysis and dichotomous data analysis that was suitable for the one-parameter Rasch model (modern probability, probability test theory, Item Response Theory, IRT method). The data was applied to the SPSS program and the R statistical ltm module.

RESULTS

I. Results of the Reliability and Validity of Our Questionnaire

The combined questions tested (n_j = *29 persons*) and retested (n_a = *27 persons*) provided the following information based on the linear correlation coefficient (Pearson's correlation coefficient) corresponding to the questions:

very high correlation, strong dependent relationship (between 0.9 – 1) in 5 questions
high correlation, marked relationship (between 0.7 - 0.9) in 8 questions
medium correlation, good relationship (between 0.4 - 0.7) in 3 questions
negligible correlation, but weak relationship (between 0.2 - 0.4) in 1 question

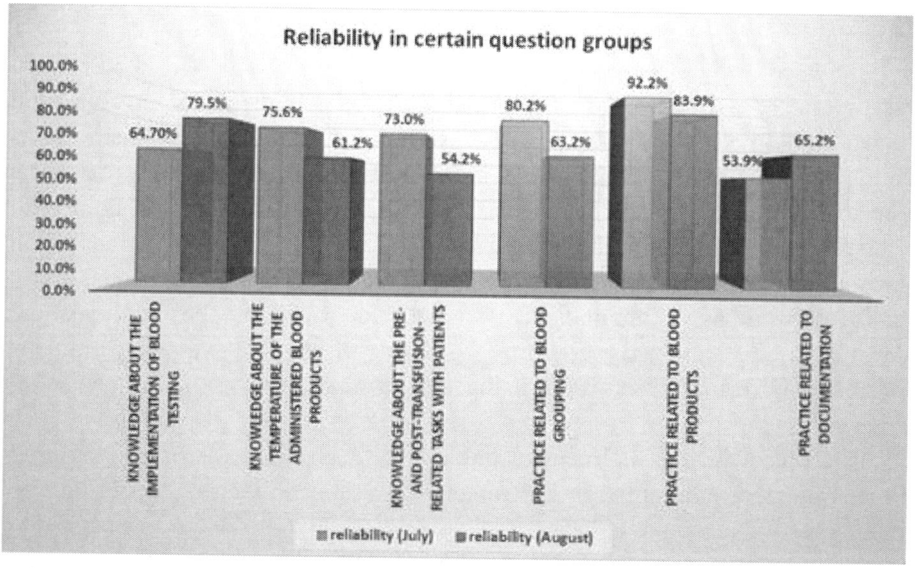

Figure 2. Reliability in certain question groups (n_j = 29, and n_a = 27).

According Cronbach alpha analysis, transfusion knowledge was 0,906 (excellent) according to the questionnaire results and was 0,880 (good) according to the re-test. In terms of transfusion therapy practice and local habit, the Cronbach alpha analysis indicated a value of 0,924 (excellent) in the questionnaire and a result of 0,894 (good) according to the retest. In reference to nursing practical skills or care functions, the Cronbach alpha analysis indicated a result of 0,969 (excellent) in the survey, and 0,953 (excellent) in the retest.

The time reliability correlation results of the survey largely indicated a strong or significant temporal reliability result, and the between the items there was a very strong and close connection.

Figure 2 summarizes some test-retest reliability measures calculated from data collected in response to selected question groups in our survey. Some questions are related to transfusion-oriented knowledge, while other items characterize transfusion practice.

II. Socio-Demographic Characteristics of the Sample in Our Nationwide Survey

657 nurses and head nurses participated in our nationwide survey from different wards from different hospitals. All returned questionnaires could be assessed. *Figure 3* shows the nurses' years in practice (n = 657 persons).

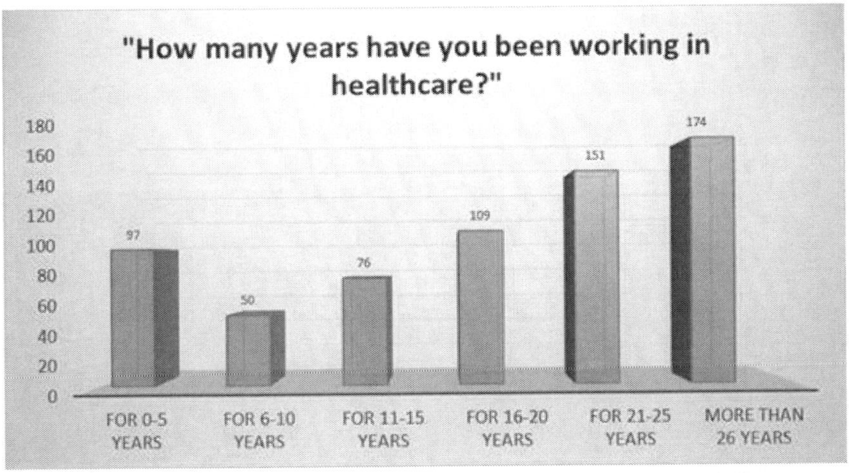

Figure 3. Nurses' years in practice.

From the whole participation sample of nurses (n = 657 persons), 478 nurses work as nurses, 123 nurses work as head nurses and 56 nurses work as a head of a unit.

Table 1 shows the frequency of the attendance of participant nurses in transfusion therapy-related tasks.

Table 1. Frequency of the attendance of participant nurses in transfusion therapy-related tasks

"How often do you have opportunity to participate in tasks related to transfusion therapy?"	
	n = 657 persons
daily	167
weekly	202
biweekly	45
monthly	69
rarely than monthly	174

Table 2. Distribution by the highest educational level

"The highest educational level"	
	n = 657 persons
vocational school	21
secondary school/ grammar school	49
"OKJ" qualification (secondary education level)	313
tertiary qualification	89
college faculty	165
university	20
PhD	-

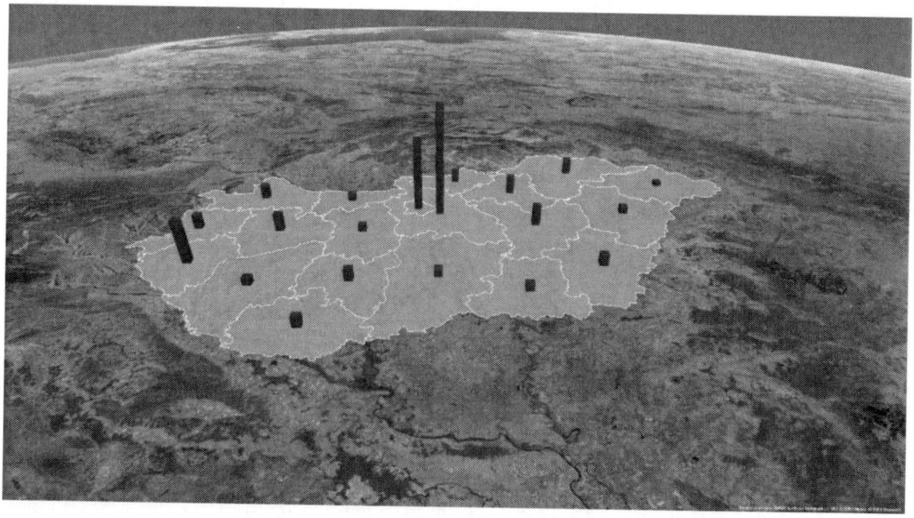

Figure 4. Distribution of workplaces by region.

Table 2 shows the distribution of the sample by the highest educational level.

147 persons attended "transfusion courses," 510 of them didn't attend "transfusion courses."

The distribution of workplaces by region was as follows (*Figure 4* and *Table 3*).

1 person didn't mark anything in relation to county.

Table 3. Distribution of workplaces by region

County	Number of the participiants
Bács-Kiskun	12
Baranya	16
Békés	17
Borsod-Abaúj-Zemplén	26
Budapest	114
Csongrád	11
Fejér	11
Győr-Moson-Sopron	23
Hajdú-Bihar	12
Heves	29
Jász-Nagykun-Szolnok	32
Komárom-Esztergom	12
Nógrád	20
Pest	171
Somogy	11
Szabolcs-Szatmár-Bereg	6
Tolna	18
Vas	22
Veszprém	27
Zala	66
Total	656

The last question from the socio-demographic questions gave participants the possibility to write multiple responses. The following responses involve the nurses work places. *Figure 5* shows the distribution of the responses.

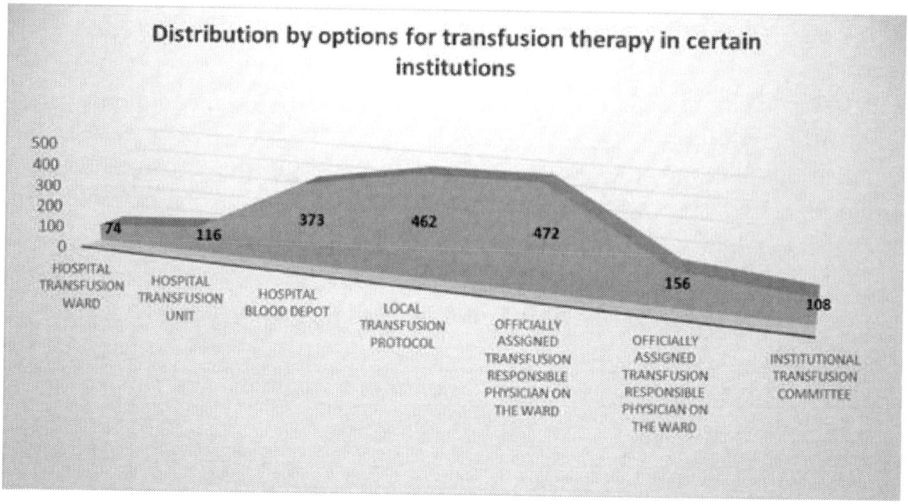

Figure 5. Distribution by options for transfusion therapy in certain institutions.

III. Results of the Knowledge-Related Questions about Transfusion Therapy and Results of the Local Practice-Related Questions about Transfusion Therapy

The test sample 42,31% (278 persons) did not know how to do blood group serology testing in terms of blood grouping nor removal of blood. 430 persons (65,45%) did not correctly know the limits of temperature for the blood before giving blood to the patient, and 213 persons (32,42%) didn't know that warmed-blood infusion has to be started immediately. 448 persons (68,19%) did not know the blood sample prior to the transfusion, whereas 444 persons (67,58%) did not know the clinical blood type determination. Except for 83 persons (12,63%) almost the entire sample group (87,36%) lacked knowledge concerning the patient's condition and corresponding transfusion indicators, aside from their lack of knowledge regarding pre-transfusion blood-group serology testing. 488 persons (74,28%) were misinformed regarding 'biological probe,' whereas 467 persons (71,08%) were not informed as to what to do after blood transfusion therapy. Within the transfusion therapy group, those who frequently (daily, weekly, bi-weekly) partook in transfusion therapy, their level of knowledge was 50,53%, whereas those nurses who rarely partook in transfusion therapy (monthly or less) resulted in a knowledge level of 51,66%.

In the nursing functions field there is also a relatively large lack of knowledge among nurses. A majority of nurses completed the following various nursing functions incorrectly: taking blood (466 persons), giving oxygen (402 persons); infusion connection (427 persons), urine sample for laboratory test (507 persons), EKG preparation (517 persons), injection administration (390 persons), medication (374 persons) and heating blood products (539 persons) (*Table 4*).

Table 4. Determination of certain nursing functions related to nursing care activities

Activity	n = 657 persons		
	I*	NI*	ID*
phlebotomy	387	191	79
measurement of the cardinal signs (blood pressure, pulse, temperature, respiration)	635	6	16
oxygen administration	238	254	165
infusion connection	199	230	228
transfusion connection	10	225	422
urine sampling for laboratory testing	461	150	46
ECG test making	466	140	51
performing of biological probe	26	271	360
patient observation	585	20	52
giving injections	238	267	152
writing of nursing documentation	646	5	6
medication administration	200	283	174
pain relief with medication	42	367	248
visits	37	100	520
blood group determination	11	289	357
heating of blood products	431	118	108

*I = independent-, NI = non-independent/dependent-, ID = interdependent nursing functions.

In the area of practical blood transfusion practices, the most problems arise in blood product heating (496 situations 75,5% of the time happens irregularly/incorrectly), the blood product connection (346 situations 75,5%-ban – takes place incorrectly), in addition, it was observed that employee duties and functions were not adequately documented (609 situation – 92,7% – inadequate documentation). The excution of the biological probe was not perfect either; the answers of 252 persons (38,35%) were incorrectly answered regarding nursing practice.

The arrival of blood products on wards are also problematic; in 114 situations (17,35%), regulations are not followed properly. Regarding transfusion therapy, nursing documentation, use and management are not unified or consistent, and in 161 (24,5%) situations, was inappropriately done. Among various institutions there are notable differences found concerning blood transfusion and therapy practices especially in regards to how nursing documentation is utilized and applied, how blood grouping is determined, as well as blood heating procedure and the instruments used to do so.

The survey indicated that 70,32%-participating nurses created his or her own hospital transfusion procedural instructions matching and taking into account the hospital's system's transfusion regulations and procedures. 23,9% ward nurses responsible for transfusions work in the wards.

IV. Results of the Use of Modern Test Theoretical Instruments

Based on the data gathered by using the Rasch practical model towards the national 'knowledge' survey, we were able to create a picture of the transfusion therapy connected questions based on the distribution of correct and incorrect answers; moreover, on the odds ratio provided a probable likelihood of the correct and incorrect answers. Based on the practical Rasch model, we created the characteristic curve which reflected the difficulty of individual items (*Figure 6* and *Figure 7*).

We further found out which questions the participants answered easily, with which they had more difficulty, and, we were able to itemize the various question combinations for which nurses typically had the correct answer.

In regards to transfusion therapy related skills and the questions concerning them, the largest ratio of nurses answered the questions concerning pre-transfusion therapy duties such as clinical AB0- and RhD blood group determination, correctly. They did this using the contributed compulsory patient information statement and consent forms. The most difficult question sets for the participants included those relating to pre-transfusion performance questions and the biological probe. These included the least correct answers. With the help of cluster analysis we were able to isolate two large categories in regards to transfusion therapy related questions upon which we could assess knowledge (*Figure 8*).

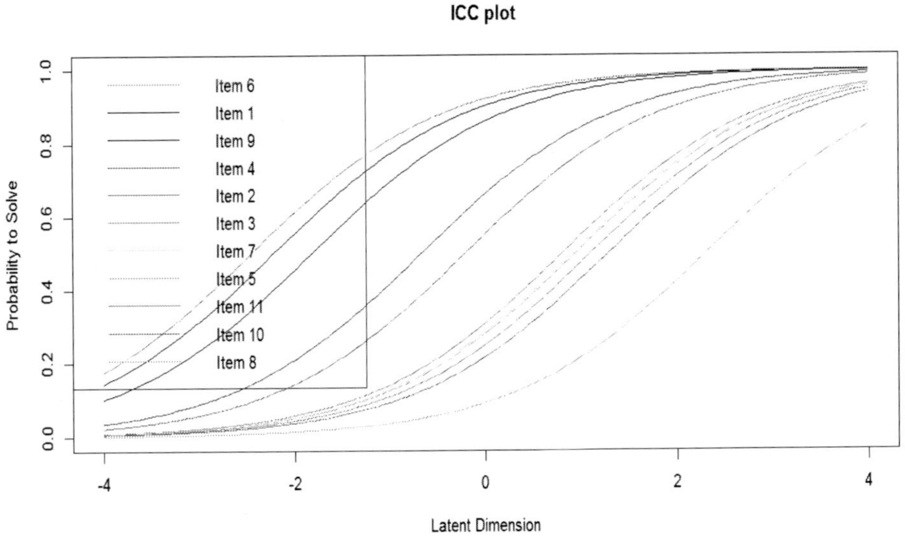

Figure 6. Items'characteristic curve in the case of questions relating to knowledge based on one-parameter Rasch model.

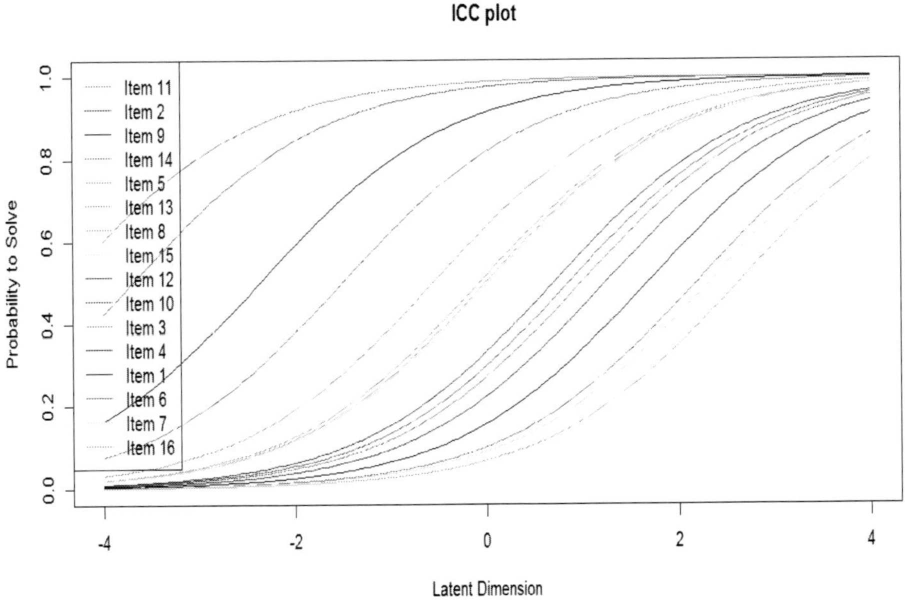

Figure 7. Items'characteristic curve in the case of nursing competencies-related knowledge based on one-parameter Rasch model.

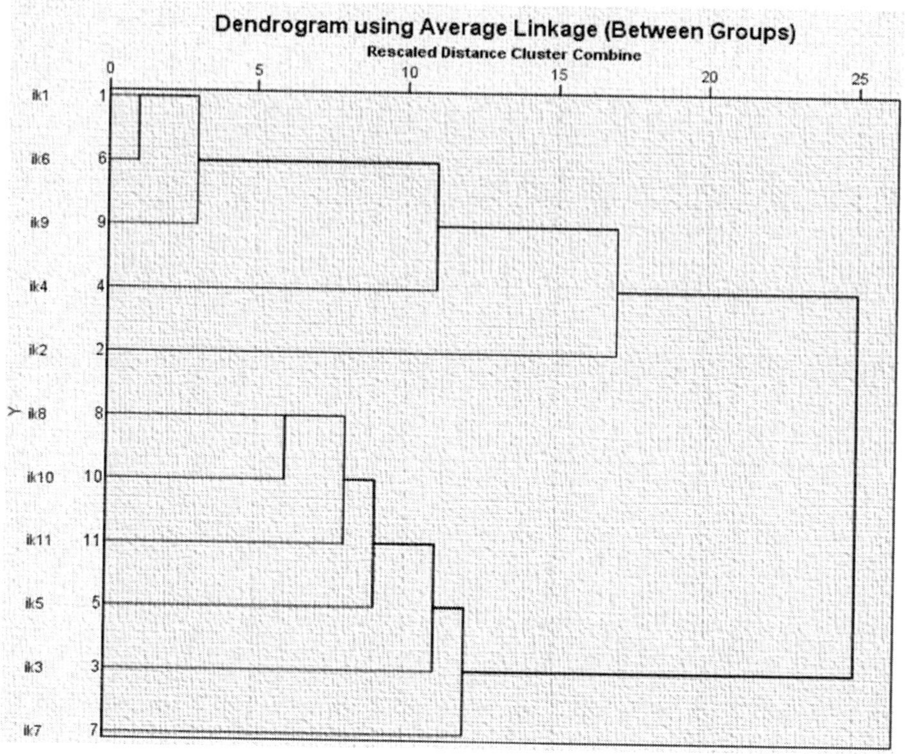

Figure 8. Dendrogram showing the transfusion therapy-related knowledge.

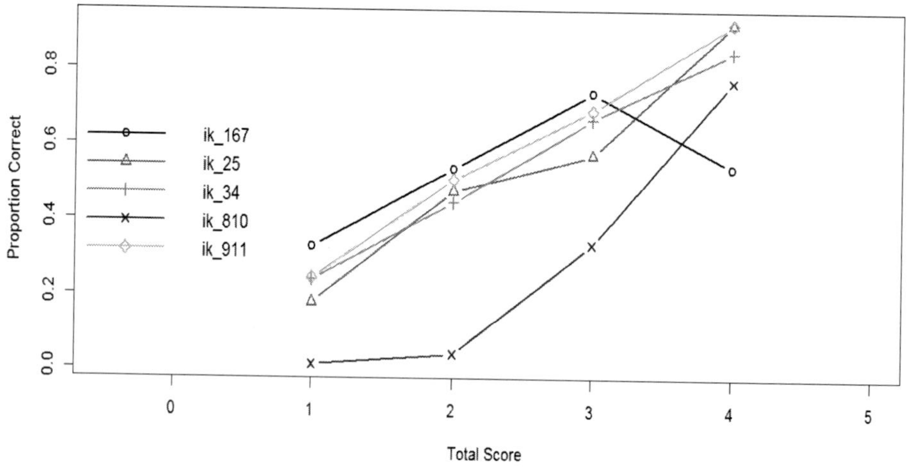

Figure 9. Distribution of correct answers per question group depending on the number of correctly answered question groups.

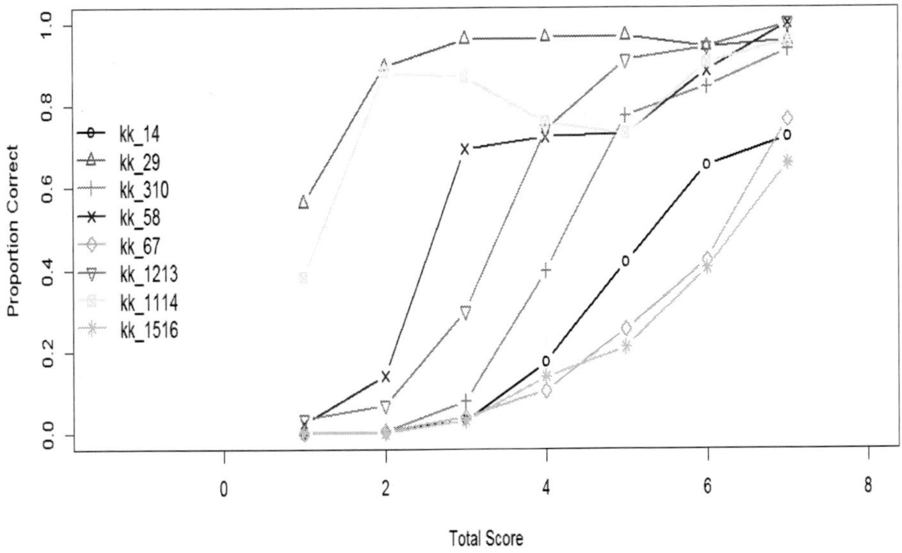

Figure 10. Distribution of correct answers per activity-pair depending on the number of correctly answered activity-pairs.

The nurses' answers regarding transfusion therapy indicated a medium performance level. Most of them could answer four, five or possibly six questions correctly out of the eleven questions provided. The 'pre-transfusion performance test plus the biological probe' question group indicated a 93% 'do not know' percentage among participants. Considering the entire question group and the answers provided by the nurses, their performance could be considered weak rather than medium level. More than one third of our sample group (39,27%) was unable to answer one correctly from the entire question groups (*Figure 9*).

The following transfusion therapy nursing competency skills were successful in ratio in that the correct determinations were made concerning nursing functions; nursing documentation management, cardinal symptoms measurement (blood pressure, pulse, temperature and breathing), and patient observation. Simultaneously, in relation to these activities, the nurses showed the least problems in terms of nursing functions and therefore these were the easiest items to answer. Overall, of the 16 nursing activities complied into 8 pairs, of the correct answer ratio per item, there was a higher ratio of improperly answered items. The nurses' performance in terms of determining nursing care activities could be considered poor because they were only able to provide correct responses to 2-3 pairs of items. Only 9 nurses (1,37%) were able to correctly determine all the activity function pairs. The greatest lack of knowledge observed among the participants was in regards to blood grouping and blood warming procedures (*Figure 10*).

Using cluster analysis we were able to categorize two large groups in terms of nursing competencies (*Figure 11*).

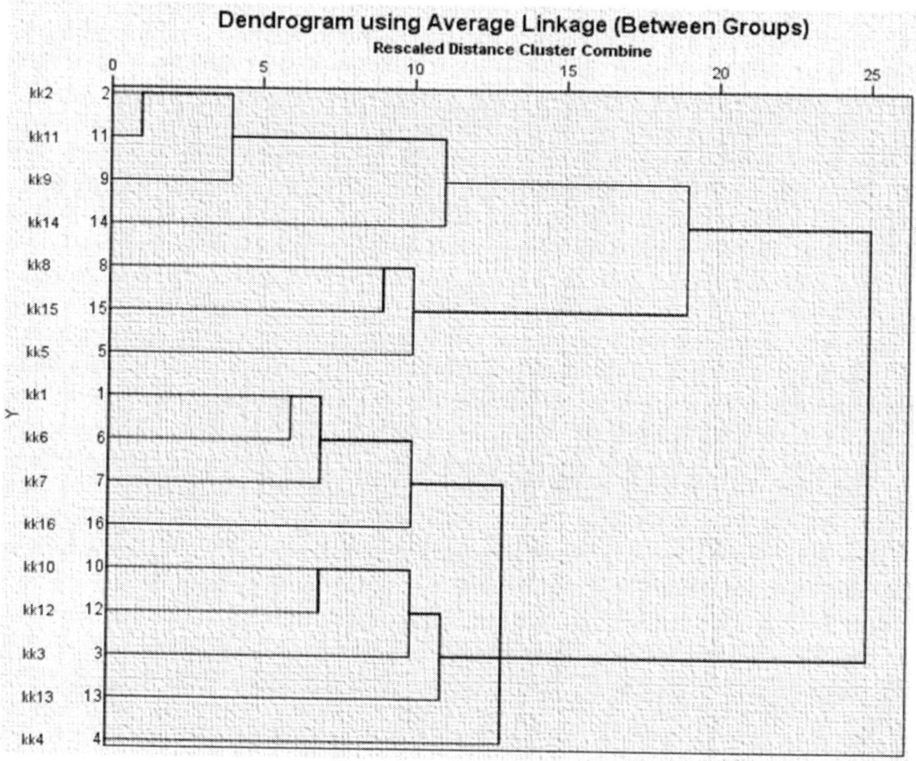

Figure 11. Dendrogram showing the knowledge about determining of nursing functions.

Discussion

In reference to the results of our survey, important differences between institutions were found in terms of transfusion therapy practice and the management of relevant documents concerning nursing duties.

1. Based on a cross-analysis of professional transfusion therapy's legal and ethical competencies, and data pooled from contingency tables, we found no substantial difference between nurses' proficiency levels and the frequency of nurses' participation in transfusion therapy.
2. Approximately ¾ (70,32%) of the institutions follow their own protocol in regards to transfusion therapy.
3. On hospital wards, approximately one fifth (23,9%) of the working nurses are certified in transfusions.
4. Based on obtained results, we found it worrying that transfusion related skills among nurses was lacking (48,905%).
5. It is in our opinion that it is equally worrying that the national institutions' typical practices are irregular or contravene regulations (as was indicated in the pilot study and national survey).
6. The ratio of nurses' lack of knowledge is unacceptably high (47,7%) as is the organization of nursing duties.
7. It is likewise unacceptable that the Transfusion Policy/Regulations were neither known nor it's criteria met.
8. With the use of modern testing instruments, objective measurements were realized.
9. Having used probabilistic methods while conducting our research, we have clearly demonstrated significant shortcomings in nurses' transfusion knowledge.

In regards to the survey we also realized certain goals.

The solution to the problems uncovered in the nursing profession lies in: increasing nurses' responsibilities, increasing the degree and the regular monitoring of aspects of transfusion therapy by head nurses, as well as, by increasing the corresponding transfusiology training and providing regular supplementary training to nurses.

CONCLUSION

New findings of our survey:

1. Our survey (N_{to} = *657*) was basically exploratory, and although there were only 657, but strong, samples, this number is representative of our national scenario of all active nurses. The relatively limited data

obtained from online research, however, was carefully and rigorously evaluated and analyzed with the intention of raising awareness.

2. We have confirmed that in regard to nurses' transfusion therapy evaluations, independent dependent and interdependent nursing competence reports are inconsistent or inharmonious.
3. Earlier national nation-wide studies were likewise not conducted among nurses in regards to transfusion therapy.
4. We initiated an objective knowledge measurement instrument using cluster analysis and multidimensional scaling in research relating to nursing science → the second survey likewise highlighted shortcomings as well as, we hope, provided new relevant information.
5. Using modern test-theory instruments we were able to realize and accomplish objective measurements.
   - we could actually determine the concrete knowledge related to transfusion therapy among nurses,
   - we could determine the nurses' abilities,
   - we could establish the degree of difficulty of the tasks and questions,
   - we were able to create a picture of the transfusion related questions through the distribution of received correct and incorrect answers,
   - furthermore, from these, the calculated logit and odds ratio were based on the possibilities of correct-incorrect responses.

REFERENCES

[1] Australian Red Cross Blood Service. Handbook for Transfusion Practitioners 2010. 2014.07.22. Available from: URL: http://resources.transfusion.com.au/cdm/singleitem/collection/p16691coll1/id/19/rec/1.

[2] Bielefeldt, S, Dewitt, J. The rules of transfusion: Best practices for blood product administration. *American Nurse Today*, 2009 2, 27-30.

[3] Boyce, N. & Brook, C. 'Towards Better, Safer Blood Transfusion.' 2015.01.21. Available from: URL: http://docs.health.vic.gov.au/docs/doc/8C312BB358B9378DCA2578E30022218A/$FILE/better-safer-transfusion.pdf.

[4] Briggs, L, Davis, R, Gutierrez, A, Kopetsky, M, Young, K, Veeramani, R. RFID in the Blood Supply Chain -- increasing productivity, quality and patient safety. *J Healthc Inf Manag*., 2009 4, 54-63.

[5] Csapó, B. Tudásszintmérő tesztek. In: F. I, Editor. *Bevezetés a pedagógiai kutatás módszereibe*. Budapest, Műszaki Tankönyvkiadó, 2000; 277–316.

[6] Csóka, M, Vingender, I. A szimulátoros oktatás módszertana. *Nővér*, 2010 6, 22-39.

[7] Dzik, WH. Transfusion safety in the hospital. *Transfusion*, 2003 43, 1190-99.

[8] Falus, I., & Ollé, J. (2007) Az empirikus kutatások gyakorlata. Adatfeldolgozás és statisztikai elemzés. Felsőoktatási tankönyv. Budapest. Nemzeti Tankönyvkiadó; 2007.

[9] Gray, A. & Melchers R. Transfusion nurses – the way forward (serious hazards of transfusion annual report 2001–2002). 2015.01.26. Available from: URL: www.shotuk.org.

[10] Jain, A. & Kaur, R. (2012). Hemovigilance and blood safety. Asian J Transfus Sci., 6(2).

[11] Jimenez-Marco, T, Clemente-Marin, G, Girona-Llobera, E, Sedeño, M, Muncunill, J. A lesson to learn from Hemovigilance: The impact of nurses'transfusion practice on mistransfusion. *Transfusion and Apheresis Science*, 2012 47, 49–55.

[12] Molnár, Gy. A Rasch-modell alkalmazása a társadalomtudományi kutatásokban. *Iskolakultúra*, 2006 12, 99-107.

[13] Molnár, Gy. Az ismeretek alkalmazásának vizsgálata modern tesztelméleti (IRT) eszközökkel. *Magyar Pedagógia*, 2003 4, 423–446.

[14] Molnár, Gy. Az objektív mérés lehetősége: a Rasch-modell. *Iskolakultúra*, 2005 3, 71-77.

[15] Nollet, KE. International trends in transfusion therapy. *Transfus Apher Sci*., 2012 1, 5-6.

[16] Nursing and Midwifery Council. Standards for medicines management. 2015.01.26. Available from: URL: http://www.nmc-uk.org/Documents/NMC-Publications/NMC-Standards-for-medicines-management.pdf.

[17] Országos Vérellátó Szolgálat. Transzfúziós szabályzat: az OVSZ módszertani levele 2. kiad. 2014.05.10. Available from: URL: http://www.ovsz.hu/sites/ovsz.hu/files/kepzes/szakmai_anyagok/transzfuzios_szabalyzat_2._kiadas/transzf_szab_2.pdf.

[18] Royal College of Nursing. Right blood, right patient, right time - Royal College of Nursing guidance for improving transfusion practice, 2013.

2014.07.28. Available from: URL: http://www.rcn.org.uk/__data/assets/pdf_file/0009/78615/002306.pdf.

[19] SHOT. Lessons for Clinical Staff from the 2007 SHOT Report. 2014.05.12. Available from: URL: http://www.shotuk.org/wp-content/uploads/2010/03/SHOT-lessons-for-clinical-staff-website.pdf.

[20] Sorra, J, Nieva, V, Fastman, BR, Kaplan, H, Schreiber, G, King, M. Staff attitudes about event reporting and patient safety culture in hospital transfusion services. *Transfusion*, 2008 9, 1934-42.

[21] Stainsby, D, Jones H, Asher D et al. Serious Hazards of Transfusion: A Decade of Hemovigilance in the UK. *Transfus Med Rev.*, 2006 4, 273-82.

[22] Weiss, Adams K, Tolich, D. Blood Transfusion: The Patient's Experience. *Am J Nurs.*, 2011 9, 24-30.

[23] WHO. Haemovigilance. 2016.04.08. Available from: URL: http://www.who.int/bloodsafety/haemovigilance/en/.

[24] Wolf, Z. R.; Hughes, R. G. (2008). Error Reporting and Disclosure. In H. R. G, Editor. *Patient Safety and Quality: An Evidence-Based Handbook for Nurses* (1st edition, 1-40). Rockville, ST: Agency for Healthcare Research and Quality.

[25] Xinming, A., Yiu-Fai, Y. Item Response Theory: What It Is and How You Can Use the IRT Procedure to Apply It. 2015.01.25. Available from: URL: https://support.sas.com/resources/papers/proceedings14/SAS364-2014.pdf.

In: Blood Donations
Editor: Antoinette Luna
ISBN: 978-1-63485-457-3

Chapter 5

A Quantitative/Qualitative Approach to Better Understand the Donation Motivations of Apheresis Donors in Quebec, Canada

Johanne Charbonneau**, Marie-Soleil Cloutier and Balia Fainstein
Research Chair of Social Aspect of Blood Donation
INRS Urbanisation Culture Société
Montreal, QC, Canada

Abstract

It is important to acquire a better understanding of the motivations of apheresis blood donors, especially in a voluntary and non-remunerated context. In 2014, we conducted a questionnaire-based survey in order to compare whole-blood donors' motivations for donating blood to those of plasma and platelet donors. To better interpret the responses provided in this study, we then conducted semi-structured qualitative interviews with 50 PPDs. For the first study, 795 whole-blood donors and 473 apheresis donors filled out a questionnaire in which they were asked to provide their motivations for donating blood. Descriptive statistics were carried out. An analysis of variance (ANOVA) was completed to determine

* Corresponding author: johanne.charbonneau@ucs.inrs.ca.

which motivators strike out between the two groups. For the second study, 50 PPDs were invited to comment on the five answer choices retained in the questionnaire-based survey. A classification grid was created, based on the 22 items proposed to respondents as motivations for donating blood. 80% of all respondents selected "My blood can save lives" in their motivators' list. When comparing results, 12 motivators are shown to be statistically different between WBDs and PPDs. For example, 61% of PPD respondents chose "Helping other people is in my nature" as one of their five most important motivators. Almost half of them also selected "I think there is a strong need for blood products" (47%) and "It gives me a sense of pride" (45%) as major motivators. The results of the interview survey suggest, for example, that the most frequently selected motivator ("My blood can save lives") has been related to many situations. Among them: 1) Being directly informed by the Blood collection agency's staff of the potential use of blood transfusions, 2) Knowing someone who has received blood transfusions, 3) Having a rare and sought-after blood type, or, 4) Having received this information from a family member who is also a blood donor. While being motivated to donate blood because "My blood can save lives" is usually interpreted as a prosocial motivation (altruism), the underlying situations rather evoke: a marketing communication strategy (1), indirect reciprocity (2), an expectation of recognition (3), or a social norm (descriptive norm) (4). A detailed analysis revealed that blood donor motivations are more complex than existing studies demonstrate. Our study is the first to combine a quantitative and qualitative approach, thereby providing a much more detailed look at PPDs' motivations for donating blood.

1. Introduction

Recruitment to the plasmapheresis panel is a crucial issue for blood collection agencies (BCAs). The demand for plasma-derived therapeutic products—particularly polyvalent intravenous immune globulin (IVIg)—is projected to increase in the future [1, 2]. However, apheresis components (plasma, platelets) are still procured from compensated donors in many high-income countries, such as Germany and the United States [3]. As is the case in many countries, in the province of Québec (Canada), the organization responsible for blood product supply, Héma-Québec, is attempting to increase its degree of self-sufficiency by appealing to non-remunerated volunteer donors [4]. From 2014 to 2015, the rate of IVIg self-sufficiency, based on non-remunerated donations, was 14.6% [5] in Québec. At a recent conference organized by Héma-Québec, national and international experts and stakeholders stated that an objective of 30% self-sufficiency was needed [5]. There are currently seven permanent collection sites equipped for apheresis donation in the province. Among them, five are equipped to collect plasmapheresis donations. According to its most recent annual report, Héma-Québec will open new permanent blood centers devoted to the collection of plasma for fractionation in the next few years. A collection program for plasma by apheresis intended for fractionation will also be extended to all permanent donor centers. There are plans for a fractionation plant to open in 2019 [6].

Apheresis donation differs in many ways from whole blood donation. In Québec, although a whole blood donor may donate once every 56 days, a plasma donor may donate every 6 days, and a platelet donor, every 14 days. In addition, plasma and platelet donation processes last longer due to the return of saline and red blood cells (RBC) to the donor: a minimum of 45 minutes for plasmapheresis and up to three hours for plateletpheresis as compared to up to 15 minutes for whole blood donation. The introduction of the possibility of collecting plasma concurrently with each platelet donation accounted for a large portion of the increase in plasma volumes collected in Québec over the last few years.

Despite the obvious need to recruit more apheresis donors, there is very little literature on the motivations of such donors. The meta-analysis review produced by Bednall and Bove in 2011 [7] on self-reported motivators for donating blood showed that only 7 studies out of 92 included plasma or platelet donors. All of the studies, but one, were conducted in countries where remuneration for plasmapheresis or plateletpheresis is available.

Analyses of apheresis donors have focused primarily on their socio-economic profile [8-10], the conversion process from whole blood to apheresis donation [7, 11-14], the barriers (deterrents) they face or their reasons for discontinuing the practice [10, 15-18], and, of course, the motivations of such donors [7-9, 19-26]. Some researchers focused on the reasons behind their first-time apheresis donation, while others also explored general motivations (or the benefits donors perceived [7]). Only three studies compared the motivations of apheresis donors with those of whole blood donors [9, 19, 24]. Out of the eleven studies on apheresis donors' motivations, three singled out platelet donors, the others concerned plasma donors. Also, three were conducted in countries where remuneration for apheresis in available; payment was then the chief motivator [8, 23, 25].

Among the studies on apheresis donors' motivations conducted in a voluntary non-remunerated (VNR) context, only two used a questionnaire-based survey. The number of answer choices given to participants [19, 24] was quite limited (6 and 9) in their case. In the Glynn et al. study [19], the most commonly reported reason to donate was "Felt it was the right thing to do." In the Veldhuizen and Dongen study [24], both whole blood and plasma donors chose "helping others" as their main reason for donating blood; it should be noted that more plasma donors than whole blood donors chose this particular motivation.

In smaller surveys, researchers chose to study motivations via semi-structured interviews or focus groups [7, 9, 20, 22, 26]. In qualitative studies, blood donation was associated with numerous motivators, including personality traits, social influences, and the sort of practical accommodations agencies are able to provide donors with. Specific motivators related to the apheresis donation were noted, such as the ease of developing a routine (due to the possibility of making an appointment), or the ability to increase the number of donations one can make. Some studies also highlighted the importance of the interpersonal relationships developed with collection staff and other donors [7, 9, 20, 22].

In the studies selected by Bednall and Bove [7] as well as in the others we found, the motivators most frequently cited by plasma and platelet donors were "prosocial." In order to produce their meta-analysis review, Bednall and Bove developed a taxonomy based on established terminology from both the psychology [27] and marketing [28] literature. They defined the "prosocial motivation" category as follows: "the desire to have a positive impact on other people or social collectives through blood donation without regard for social or material rewards" (p. 320). Such motivators could be associated to collectivism ("To help the community") as much as they are to altruism ("I enjoy helping others"). But what exactly does the blood donor means when he says he donates because he enjoys helping others? What is behind this?

Interpreting the exact meaning behind the answers chosen by respondents as motivations for donating blood can be difficult. The notion of altruism illustrates this quite well. When analysing the way this notion was used by various researchers, it is clear they disagree on its definition [29-31]. In the previously cited study by Glynn et al. [32] the "Felt it was the right thing to do" statement used in their 1998 questionnaire was specifically chosen as a measure of altruism in a list of nine reasons that could potentially have motivated individuals the last time they donated. Eighty percent of respondents chose this statement from the list, leading the researchers to conclude that altruism was the main reason why people donate blood. In the following years, the results of this study were used and cited by countless researchers [4, 33-38] despite the fact that it is obviously difficult to know how the respondents would themselves define the notion of altruism. Furthermore, the particular statement chosen by Glynn et al. [32] illustrates both the idea of duty and obligation as well as of a free and voluntary act [10, 39], which is generally associated with blood donation. Later researchers would interpret the idea with a focus on the idea of duty and obligation [37, 38].

Other examples also demonstrate how difficult it can be to interpret the meaning of brief and rather vague statements used in survey questionnaires to find out about blood donors' motivations. For example, "personal recognition" [7] may belong as much in the "social norms" category, if friends and family members express such recognition, as in the "incentives" category, if it comes from BCAs instead. "Wishing to increase one's number of donations"—an item very popular among apheresis donors—may itself be interpreted as an "intrinsic" motivator ("need […] which arises from within the individual and causes action toward some *goals*"), that could be highly influenced by the "recognition" mechanisms established by BCAs to express gratefulness toward their most frequent donors (certificate, badges, awards' events).

In short, the studies discussed thus have numerous limitations. As noted by Bednall and Bove [7], few researchers have attempted to study apheresis donation in the context of VNR donation. Analysis of motivations has often been limited in scope, due either to the restricted number of answer choices provided, or to the researcher's decision to focus on the primary motivator. Qualitative studies may help better interpret the motivations of apheresis donors, but they too have limitations, due to the difficulty of generalizing results. To our knowledge, no study to date on PPDs' motivations for donating blood in a VNR context has ever combined a questionnaire-based survey with a full qualitative approach, using semi-structured interviews rather than only open-ended questions within a questionnaire.

This chapter aims to better understand the motivations of regular plasma/platelet donors (PPDs) in a voluntary and non-remunerated context by combining quantitative and qualitative approaches. In 2014, we conducted a questionnaire survey in order to compare whole-blood donors' motivations for donating blood to those of plasma and platelet donors. To better interpret the responses provided by apheresis donors in this study, we then conducted semi-structured qualitative interviews with 50 PPDs. This study seeks to provide a thorough analysis of the motivations of PPDs by combining the results of the two studies.

2. Materials and Methods

a. Questionnaire-Based Survey (QBS)

Sample Selection

Sampling was done by accessing and extracting information from Héma-Québec's donor information system (Progesa). Since 1987, this computerized database has included personal information on date of birth, gender, address of residence, dates of all previous donations, types of donations, previous and current deferrals, and screening test results for all donors. Two[1] groups of donors were defined on the basis of their donation history: current whole-blood donors (WBD) were those who had given 2 allogenic donations during their previous history and 1 donation during the six months preceding the survey; and plasma and platelet donors (PPD) were those who had given 3 plasma or platelet donations during their previous history and 1 during the six months preceding the survey. Age (between 18 and 55 years-old) and gender (women were over-sampled for PPD, since they are less often donors) were also taken into account.

The initial targeted number of respondents was 750 subjects (50% men, 50% women): 500 regular WBDs and 250 regular PPDs. To achieve this target, 2000 WBDs were randomly selected from the database. The Progesa database contained only 1968 donors who met our criteria (453 women and 1515 men) for the selection of PPDs. From this pool, all the women were selected and 547 men were randomly selected. Sampling was conducted on March 25, 2014. Full details of the methodology, questionnaire development, and survey procedures used are provided elsewhere [40].

Questionnaire Development

Data were collected using a self-administered mailed questionnaire developed specifically for the study (available upon request to the authors). The final version of the questionnaire consisted of 25 questions and took approximately 20 minutes to complete. Two separate questionnaires were produced: one for the WBDs, and one for the PPDs, where subjects were asked if they would like to participate in a qualitative follow-up survey.

---

[1] A third group of lapsed donors was also recruited for this survey but was not used in the present analysis.

Table 1. Question on Motivators for Donating Blood

Time use and blood donation questionnaire Question 1 "Which of the following elements motivate you to donate blood? (Check off up to five answers)"	References	Motivator categories (Bednall and Bove [7])
A blood drive is being held near where I live or near my workplace / place of study	[15, 43, 65]	Convenience of collection site
		Prosocial motivation
My blood can save lives	[21, 43, 46, 47, 60]	Altruism
It's a positive thing to do and requires little effort	[9, 22, 35, 43, 65]	Altruism
It's my civic duty/It's a way to help out the community	[21, 22, 35, 43, 44, 49, 52, 61, 65, 66]	Collectivism (community)
I give thinking that a member of my family or a close friend could need blood someday	[20, 24, 43, 65, 67]	Collectivism (family/ friends)
		Personal values
Helping other people is in my nature	[22, 35, 43, 44, 49, 61]	Personal moral norms
My religious practice or convictions have encouraged me to donate	[22, 43, 49]	Religiosity
I think there is a strong need for blood products	[9, 22, 43, 45, 49, 52, 65, 66]	Perceived need for donation
		Indirect reciprocity
Someone close to me has received one or more blood transfusions in the past	[7, 21, 22, 24, 43, 45, 52, 65]	Upstream
It gives me confidence that others will give if I need it later	[20, 21, 43, 65, 67]	Downstream
I like to have goals (20, 50, 100, 200 donations, etc.)	[21, 43, 45]	Intrinsic motivation
It gives me a sense of pride	[22, 24, 35, 43, 45]	Self-esteem
		Marketing communication
I receive telephone reminders from Héma-Québec	[43, 49, 56-58]	Direct marketing
When I see posters and advertising	[43, 49]	Advertising
I join people that I know (donors, staff) at the blood drive	[16, 17, 20, 22, 43, 45]	Blood drives
		Incentives
It's an activity that encourages you to monitor and take care of your health	[43, 45, 49]	Perceived health benefits
It gives me energy in the following days	[9, 35, 43, 66]	
I have a rare and sought-after blood type	[43, 61, 65, 68]	Learn blood type
I feel recognition from people around me	[22, 43, 45]	Recognition
		Social norms
Blood donation is a tradition in my family	[20, 22, 43, 45, 67]	Descriptive norm
My coworkers also give blood	[43, 49, 67]	Subjective norm
I like to be accompanied	[20, 43]	Subjective norm
Other reason (specify):		

The first question concerned motivators for blood donation. Several sources were used in selecting and formulating the proposed answer choices (see Table 1). Respondents were given the opportunity to check off the five answers out of 22 that they consider relevant when asked about their motives for donating blood. They were also permitted to add their own reasons. They were not, however, asked to indicate a chief motive or rate their answers.

Survey Procedures and Data Analysis

An introductory letter signed by an executive officer at Héma-Québec was included in the mailing package, along with a letter explaining the study signed by the head researcher, the questionnaire, the consent form, and a pre-stamped return envelope. Questionnaires were mailed based on the language preference information provided in the donor information system (French, 2868; English, 130). Questionnaires were anonymous (no individual identifiers retained) but return envelopes were supplied with a code, permitting the questionnaire to be tracked back to the original database. Ethics approvals were delivered by both the university center and Héma-Québec. The questionnaire mail-out began on April 25, 2014. The last completed questionnaire was received on January 28, 2015.

A total of 1361 were returned fully or partially completed and 1268 questionnaires were admissible for the analysis. The response rate was 40% for the WBD group (795/2000) and 48% for the PPD group (473/1000). As has been found elsewhere [41, 42], response rates were higher among women, especially for WBDs (46% versus 34% for men). Older donors (50-56 years old) had the highest response rates (11% for WBDs and 15% for PPDs) while the 30- to 39-year-old group had the lowest response rates both for WBDs (8%) and PPDs (9%). Differences with other age groups were small.

b. Semi-Structured Qualitative Interviews with Apheresis Donors (SSQI)

Complex social behaviour, such as blood donation, is influenced by a variety of factors that cannot always be categorized or ranked by order of importance without losing part of its richness [43, 44]. The purpose of the interviews was that of analysing apheresis donors' motivations and practices in detail.

Sample Selection

The targeted number of respondents was 50 subjects. As in the previous study, plasma and platelet donors (PPDs) were those who had given 3 plasma or platelet donations during their previous history and 1 during the 6 months preceding the survey. Gender (50% men, 50% women) was also taken into account. It was important to interview people from contrasting categories. Accordingly, the research team decided to conduct interviews in three different cities: Montréal (20), Québec city (20) and Trois-Rivières (10). The permanent collection site dedicated to plasmapheresis donations in Trois-Rivières is among the most recently opened in Québec (in 2014). In the QBS, we chose to restrict our study to donors between the ages of 18 and 55. This survey also aimed to better understand how women in their thirties and forties integrated blood donation into their daily lives, what barriers they experienced and the reasons they discontinued the practice. This is precisely why this sample was age-specific. However, a demographic report on blood donors produced by Héma-Québec (2014–2015) showed that 47% of apheresis donors in Québec were 50 years of age and over (60% in the Montreal area). Analyses conducted in other countries [21, 45] reported similar results: a higher proportion of older, retirement-aged donors (mostly men) are active in the pool of plasmapheresis donors. As a result, the research team chose to add respondents from the 56 to 70-year-old group to the qualitative study (Montréal, 5/20; Québec City, 5/20, Trois-Rivières, 4/20).

The first sample drawn on in this study was a subgroup of the QBS. PPD subjects recruited in the QBS (18 to 55-year-old group) were asked if they would like to take part in a qualitative follow-up survey. Thirty-three percent of PPD respondents (162/473) agreed to be contacted by the research team and gave their telephone number for follow-up. This group was stratified first into 3 groups (Montréal, Québec City, Trois-Rivières), then by gender (50/50) and age group (20–29, 30–39, 40–49, 50 and over). For the purpose of defining donor status, lifetime blood donation history was considered. Lifetime donation history was not only based on Progesa-recorded donations but also on all other donations reported by the donor, including those made before the computerized database was introduced. Three groups were then defined: 1) 3 to 24 donations; 2) 25 to 100 donations; 3) Over 100 donations. 36 PPDs were randomly selected to take part in the SSQI study (22%, 36/162). To complete our target and include the 56- to 70-year-old group, 120 subjects were randomly selected from the Progesa database, following the same criteria used for the 20- to 55-year-old group.

Semi-Structured Protocol

Interviews' guide was inspired by our other qualitative studies on blood donor's motivations and practices conducted in previous years [43]. The semi-structured protocol covered a broad spectrum of issues. The main topics were: 1) knowledge of blood donation before the first donation; 2) donor's motivations; 3) history of first donation (whole blood and apheresis); 4) usual blood donation practice and changes over the years; 5) demographic characteristics. To explore the donor's motivations, the research team chose to draw directly on the answers given by the respondent in the QBS. Respondents were asked to explain: 1) the reasons why they had checked off each of the five answers (out of 22) that they considered relevant when asked about motives for donating blood and, 2) the meaning given by the respondent to each selected motive.

Considering the fact that respondents recruited from the 56- to 70-year-old-group were not part of the QBS, they were specifically instructed to fill out the questionnaire (at home) before the interview.

Interview Procedures

All donors selected from the QBS were contacted by a research assistant over the phone. Because they had already agreed to take part in the follow-up survey, the assistant simply needed to re-confirm their agreement to take part, explain the new procedure and make an appointment. These respondents nevertheless received a new mailing package that included an introductory letter signed by an executive officer at Héma-Québec and the consent form. Respondents were also given an information sheet that provided some background information on the new study, described the interview process, and listed the general topics to be discussed.

Donors selected from the 56- to 70-year-old group using the Progesa database were contacted by the main researcher (first author of this chapter) over the phone. During the call, the researcher explained the study's objectives and the interview process, and then asked the donor if he or she agreed to take part in the study. All of the donors contacted in this case agreed. Before concluding the call, an appointment was made with each of the donors. These particular respondents received the same mailing package as the first group, with the addition of the questionnaire used in the QBS. They were asked to bring it with them for the interview.

All interviews were carried out in French, between August 1st and September 29th, 2014. At first, interviews were conducted with two team members present. After 6 interviews were completed in Montréal, the remaining interviews were conducted by a single interviewer (B. Fainstein, Montréal and Trois-Rivières; J. Charbonneau, Québec City). Team's discussions occurred in tandem with data collection, with key statements and themes being immediately identified and noted to inform subsequent thematic analysis.

Interviews were held either at the respondent's home, at a permanent collection center or at the research institute and lasted anywhere between 45 minutes and 2 hours. They were conducted using an anthropological approach, meaning that the grid was less structured than it would be in a regular interview. The goal was to allow respondents to describe the meanings that may have been obscured through the strict nature of the QBS.

Interview material was supplemented with handwritten notes and observations taken during the interview. These notes consisted mainly of themes identified in the course of conversation, which could require further exploration. Other notes included general information about the interview context itself. For example, whether there were any interruptions, other people present and any topics that were particularly easy or difficult to talk about.

All interviews were recorded and transcribed. Ethics approvals were delivered by both the university center and Héma-Québec and informants were asked to sign consent forms before submitting to the interview. Informants were also clearly informed of that their anonymity and confidentiality would be protected.

QBS and SSQI Data Analysis

QBS data entry on ACCESS began in July 2014. Descriptive statistics were carried out for motivations and demographic variables. Chi-two tests were completed to determine which motivations stood out across the two groups (WBDs and PPDs). Analyses were performed with SAS version 9.4.

SSQI data was analyzed manually using a classification grid. First, the team retained the following themes, which are in accordance with the interview guide's different sections: 1) donor's demographic profile; 2) blood donation history; 3) practical aspects of blood donation; 4) apheresis donation's individual and social meanings; 5) donors' motivations; 6) relational aspects of blood donation (with other donors/Héma-Québec staff); 7) institutional aspects of blood donation experience. Grid categories for donors' motivations were developed based on the 22 items offered to respondents as motivators for donating blood in the QBS (see Table 1). Brainstorming team discussions were held in order to add sub-categories that had emerged after having re-read the transcriptions. Each of the 22 items was then subdivided into specific dimensions, according to similarities between participants' answers or emphasis on specific points. Interviews were coded accordingly, line by line, re-read by the main researcher, and compared with others interviews to derive consistent themes as well as variations which point to extreme cases.

3. QBS and SSQI's Population Profiles

The final QBS sample had more women in the WBD (58% women) group, but proportions of women and men were equivalent in the PPD group, considering that we had oversampled women (Table 2). This differed from the original BCA panel of donors, where WBD proportions are more similar (46% women, 54% men) but where women represented only 22% of PPDs. On the other hand, in the apheresis BCA panel[2], women represented 45% of plasma donors. Age groups were similar for WBDs and PPDs, with 25% of respondents belonging to the 18- to 29-year-old category, respectively 22% and 19% of WBD and PPD respondents belonging to the 30- to 39-year-old category; almost a quarter of respondents to the 40- to 49-year-old category (23% for WBDs and 25% for PPDs) a third to the 50- to 56-year-old age groups (30% for WBDs and 32% for PPDs). In comparison, the original BCA database had a greater number of older donors (50 and over) among WBDs (42%) and PPDs (48%). In terms of education and marital status, both groups were well educated (between 36% and 40% of respondents had university degrees) and the majority of respondents were married (63% and 64%). We could not compare these variables with the BCA's broader panel. WBD respondents came mostly from Montréal (39% against 22% for PPDs) and elsewhere in Québec (43% against 19% for PPDs). In part due to the small number of plasmapheresis collection sites in the province at the time of this survey, most PPDs came from the Québec City area (59%). Only the gender and region of origin variables were statistically different between the two groups.

In the SSQI sample, proportions of women and men were equivalent (Table 3), as in the PPD group of the QBS. In the BCA apheresis panel, as previously mentioned, women represented 22% of PPDs and 45% of plasma donors. In the SSQI sample, there was almost the same proportion of

---

[2] The BCA apheresis panel includes donors of plasma and other products (platelets or targeted blood components).

respondents in the 20- to 29-year-old (20%), the 30- to 39-year-old (20%) and the 40- to 49-year-old age groups (18%). The decision to add a 56- to 70 year-old age group to the SSQI sample resulted in a greater number (42%) of older donors (50 and over) than in the QBS sample (31%). In this regard, the SSQI age groups distribution is closer to the BCA panel than the QBS was when it comes to the 40 years and over group. In terms of education, SSQI respondents were almost as well educated (50% Cégep[3], 34% University) as those in the QBS sample (40%/40%). The majority of respondents were married (52%) but this sample included a greater number of single respondents (38%) or divorced/separated/widowed (10%) than in the QBS sample (31%/6%). In this regard, the SSQI sample is more diverse.

Table 2. Comparison of demographic variables for WBDs and PPDs responding to the questionnaire (QBS)

	Total	%	WBDs	%	PPDs	%	*Sign. (p)*
	n = 1268		n = 795		n = 473		
Women	696	55	458	58	238	50	p < 0,05
Men	572	45	337	42	235	50	
18-29 years	317	25	200	25	117	25	n.s.
30-39 years	265	21	176	22	89	19	
40-49 years	300	24	182	23	118	25	
50-56 years	386	30	237	30	149	31	
Elementary/High School	295	23	199	25	96	20	n.s.
CÉGEP*	498	39	311	39	187	40	
University	473	37	283	36	190	40	
Single	363	29	218	28	145	31	
Married-common law	804	64	506	65	298	63	n.s.
Divorced-separated-widowed	81	7	51	7	30	6	
Respondent from the Quebec city region	419	33	141	18	278	59	p < 0,0001
Respondent from the Montreal region	416	33	311	39	105	22	
Respondent from other region	433	34	343	43	90	19	

[3] In Quebec, CEGEP (for Collège d'enseignement général et professionnel) is an educational stage between high school and university, and is comprised of professional technical programs (3 years) and general pre-university programs (2 years).

Table 3. Comparison of demographic variables for PPDs from the QBS, the SSQI and the BCA panel (2014-2015)

	QBS		SSQI		BCA panel (2014-2015)	
	PPDs	%	PPDs	%	PPDs	%
	n = 473		n = 50		n = 9915	
Women	238	50	25	50	2139	22
Men	235	50	25	50	7716	78
18-29 years	117	25	10	20	2491	25
30-39 years	89	19	10	20	1258	13
40-49 years	118	25	9	18	1389	14
50-55 years	149	31	7	14	4777	48
56 and over			14	28		
Elementary/High School	96	20	8	16		
CÉGEP	187	40	25	50		
University	190	40	17	34		
Single	145	31	19	38		
Married-common law	298	63	26	52		
Divorced-separated-widowed	30	6	5	10		
Respondent from the Quebec city region	278	59	20	40	5206	53
Respondent from the Montreal region	105	22	20	40	3631	37
Respondent from other region	90	19	10	20	1078	11

The purpose of this chapter is to provide a thorough analysis of the motivations of PPDs by combining the results of the two studies. QBS results will be presented first. Recall that this survey aimed to compare the motivations of WBDs with those of PPDs. As part of the analysis, we will focus specifically on the nature of the PPDs' motivations; a detailed comparison of these two groups has already been published [10]. For the purpose of this analysis, we also classified the motivation statements from the categories identified by Bednall and Bove [7] as part of their meta-analysis (see Table 1).

4. Results of the Questionnaire-Based Survey

Table 4 presents the proportion of respondents in the whole sample and the two sub-samples (WBDs and PPDs) that selected each of the motivators.

The motivator indicated by the highest percentage of respondents (80%) was "My blood can save lives," which was chosen by more WBDs (83%) than PPDs (77%). A comparison of WBDs and PPDs according to their reported motivators shows that results for 12 motivators were significantly different from one group to another from a statistical standpoint.

Table 4. Proportions of WBD and PPD Respondents for Each Selected Motivators

Motivators	All donors (n = 1268)	WBDs (n = 795)	PPDs (n = 473)	*P*
My blood can save lives	80%	83%	77%	<0,05
It's a positive thing to do and requires little effort	54%	62%	52%	<0,001
Helping other people is in my nature	47%	49%	61%	<0,0001
I think there is a strong need for blood products	46%	38%	47%	<0,05
I give thinking that a member of my family or a close friend could need blood someday	44%	47%	40%	<0,01
It gives me a sense of pride	35%	33%	45%	<0,0001
A blood drive is being held near where I live or near my workplace / place of study	31%	34%	8%	NS
It's my civic duty / a way to help out the community	30%	32%	28%	<0,0001
I receive telephone reminders from Héma-Québec	19%	18%	28%	<0,0001
I have a rare and sought-after blood type	16%	17%	14%	<0,0001
Someone close to me has received one or more blood transfusions in the past	15%	16%	16%	NS
It gives me confidence that others will give if I need it later	13%	12%	11%	NS
I like to have goals (20, 50, 100, 200 donations, etc.)	12%	13%	23%	NS
When I see posters and advertising	8%	5%	1%	NS
It's an activity that encourages you to monitor and take care of your health	7%	8%	9%	NS
Blood donation is a tradition in my family	7%	6%	6%	NS
Other reason	6%	6%	8%	NS
I feel recognition from people around me	5%	6%	7%	< 0,05
It gives me energy in the following days	4%	5%	3%	<0,0001
My coworkers also give blood	2%	2%	1%	<0,05
I join people that I know (donors, staff) at the blood drive	1%	1%	2%	NS
My religious practice or convictions have encouraged me to donate	1%	1%	1%	NS
I like to be accompanied	1%	1%	0%	NS

PPDs reported several motivators in greater proportions to WBDs. The "Helping other people is in my nature" (61%) motivator had the highest proportion of PPD respondents. Also, almost half of PPDs stated that "I think there is a strong need for blood products" (47%) and "It gives me a sense of pride" (45%) were important motivators. Lastly, almost a third of them choose "I receive telephone reminders from Héma-Québec" (28%) and a smaller proportion choose "I feel recognition from people around me" (7%) as one of their five most important motivators.

Table 5 presents the proportion of QBS respondents for each of Bednall and Bove's [7] motivator categories. These categories combine all of the motivators shown in Table 1. The category with the highest percentage is the "prosocial motivation," with 97% of both WBD and PPD respondents having selected at least one motivation in this category. The comparison of WBDs and PPDs according to their reported proportions of motivators in each category shows that results were significantly different from a statistical perspective for five of the categories, four of them having higher proportions for PPDs. Approximately two-thirds of PPD respondents chose motivators in the "personal values" (61%) and "indirect reciprocity" (67%) categories, having a higher proportion than WBDs for both categories (with 50% and 56% of WBDs choosing these categories respectively). Two other categories were higher for PPDs: the "perceived need for donation" (47%) and the "marketing communication" motivators (30%).

Table 5. Proportions of WBD and PPD Respondents for Each of Bednall and Bove's Motivator Categories [7]

Motivator categories*	All donors (n = 1268)	WBDs (n = 795)	PPDs (n = 473)	*P* from Khi-2
Convenience of collection sites	24%	34%	8%	< 0,0001
Prosocial motivation	97%	97%	97%	NS
Personal values	54%	50%	61%	< 0,0001
Perceived need for donation	41%	38%	47%	< 0,01
Indirect reciprocity	60%	56%	67%	< 0,0001
Marketing communication	25%	22%	30%	< 0,01
Incentives	31%	31%	29%	NS
Social norms	15%	15%	14%	NS

*See Table 1 for the list of motivators in each category.

5. Semi-Structured Qualitative Interviews Results

SSQI results are used to provide a more in-depth analysis of the meaning behind 6 motivations selected as part of the QBS: 1) the motivation most often selected by both groups (WBDs and PPDs): “My blood can save lives” and 2) the five motivations which were selected by PPDs significantly more often: “Helping others is in my nature,” “I think there is a strong need for blood products,” “It gives me a sense of pride,” “I receive telephone reminders from Héma-Québec “ and “I like to have goals.”

“My Blood Can Save Lives”

In the QBS, 77% of PPD respondents reported this statement to explain why they gave blood. In the SSQI study, 35 respondents (out of 50) also selected it. As in the QBS, it was the most frequently selected motivator. This particular item is usually regarded as a prosocial altruistic motivation [22, 46, 47]. Bednall and Bove [7] defined a “prosocial motivation” as “the desire to have a positive impact on other people […] through blood donation without regard for social or material rewards” (p. 320). In this category, altruism is a “motivation with the ultimate goal of increasing the welfare of one or more individuals (especially strangers) through blood donation without a regard for social or material reward.” (p.320) This motivation refers to one of the key ethical principles outlined by Beauchamp and Childress [48], benevolence, which can be defined as an act performed for the well-being of others. In other words “a moral obligation to do good and act with the best intentions towards others.” (p. 201) Rules of benevolence identified by these authors include that of rescuing those in danger. This, of course, applies perfectly to the idea of blood donation, which essentially helps “save lives.” In a study carried out in 1998, Fernandez-Montoya classified this statement along with those associated to “awareness of a concrete need.” On the basis of this interpretation, this statement should actually be classified in the “perceived need for donation” category proposed by Bednall and Bove. But, what does it really mean? What exactly are the donors referring to when choosing this statement to explain the reasons why they give blood?

According to SSQI data analysis, this most frequently chosen motivator has been interpreted in a variety of different ways by the respondents.

It may very well take on the general meaning of prosocial altruistic motivator aimed at improving the well-being of others (strangers). "I truly feel that, whether its red blood cells, white blood cells or plasma, it can truly save lives." (Female, 51 years old, Montréal, 33 donations). The donor imagines a person in need, but does not refer to any concrete situation. "I know that when the person at the other end receives the blood, I am saving a life or helping him get better." (Female, 47 years old, Montréal, 76 donations) "I do it to help others, for children. If it can help save lives, then I think that's great." (Female, 31 years old, Trois-Rivières, 7 donations). Other respondents make reference to more specific health problems (cancer, accident victims): "There are often accidents and things like that." (Female, 49 years old, Montréal, 7 donations)

> Somebody somewhere is going to get this blood. At least, I imagine so. I always tell myself it could be anyone. Someone who is really sick, has leukemia or something like that, and really needs this blood to survive [...]. I guess when you need a blood donation, it's generally a life or death thing... isn't it? (Female, 22 years old, Montréal, 25 donations)

This way of explaining one's motivation to "save lives" by giving blood can be considered an altruistic motivation. However, this is true insofar as it is combined with one's knowledge of the *need for blood products*. One might have gained this knowledge by witnessing situations, whether at work (hospital setting) or elsewhere (accident, for example) that truly support the idea that "giving blood saves lives."

> I volunteered at the hospital's palliative care unit [...] I was in the unit responsible mainly for treating people with cancer, leukemia, so there were people there who constantly needed blood. [...] I witnessed people's anguish when they needed blood and there was none available to give them [...] That's when I told myself it was important to give. (Female, 70 years old, Montréal, 200 + donations)

In certain cases, the targeted needs expressed by certain donors give the impression that they are focusing on their own sense of pride. "I have a rare blood type. [...] I would tell myself I was giving because my blood type was rare [...] I would see sick kids, people who really needed it." (Female, 55 years old, Montréal, 180 donations) This particular argument hints at a desire for *indirect reciprocity* (*self-esteem*). "My blood type is B negative. They told me that there are kids who really needed it. It seemed like there was an urgent need for my blood type. I was happy to hear them say 'we need it'; it boosts your spirits even more when they tell you that." (Male, 66 years old, Trois-Rivières, 18 donations)

Certain respondents added that they were aware that the BCA was forced to import plasma-derived products from abroad or that they knew that plasma or platelet donations could help more people and therefore help "save *more* lives.[45]" "I remember seeing a Héma-Québec leaflet that mentioned it could help more people." (Male, 21 years old, Montréal, 5 donations) "Because I am a platelet donor, I saw that it could help people with cancer live longer." (Male, 26 years old, Québec City, 124 donations) These more technical arguments, used by certain respondents to explain why they chose "My blood can save lives" as one of the items offered in the QBS, demonstrates the influence of the BCA's *communication strategies*. Blood donation staff members are the ones who provide this information to the blood donors. "Your body contains 5 liters of blood, so you can save 5 lives […]. That's what they told us. One particular nurse I knew […] always explained things to us, taught us all about it, and told us how it was." (Female, 69 years old, Québec City, 386 donations)

From a general perspective, it can be noted that the association between blood donation and the gift of life is the most recurrent element in the rhetorical discourse of BCAs. "Héma-Québec tells us that a single blood donation can save 4 lives." (Male, 26 years old, Québec City, 124 donations) "Of course, the ads tend to focus on that." (Female, 49 years old, Québec City, 89 donations) This motivation, encouraged by BCAs, spotlights the value of blood, which, indeed, serves to save lives. "It saves lives. It's a fact." (Male, 30 years old, Québec City, 65 donations)

Other respondents explain that their blood donation can "save lives" because people around them, who are also blood donors, have told them so. "My niece was explaining that platelets only live 5 days. And, if you need platelets in an emergency situation, you just can't wait around. So, it's really useful." (Female, 59 years old, Montréal, 195 donations) This explanation illustrates how this motivation can be associated to the category of *social norms* (*descriptive norms*), which emphasizes how other people influence the practice of blood donation.

Lastly, this motivation can also be inspired by personal experience. For example, when the life of a loved one was saved through a blood transfusion: "[The triggering event was] my son's operation. Everything went well, the doctors were pleased, and he is doing really well now […] the pediatricians said he had needed lots of blood." (Female, 65 years old, Trois-Rivières, 8 donations) This particular argument leads us to classify this motivation under the *indirect reciprocity* (*upstream*) category.

In short, "My blood can save lives" as a reason for donating blood is clearly, for certain donors, a prosocial altruist motivation. However, because the explanations offered by the respondents also included other interpretations, this motivation could also be associated with categories such as: 1) perceived need for donation; 2) indirect reciprocity; 3) marketing communications, and 4) social norms.

Will the interpretation of the "Helping others is in my nature" item prove to be as varied?

"Helping Others Is in My Nature"

In the QBS (61%) and in the SSQI (32/50), this is the second most frequently selected motivator among respondents (32/50), ranking behind "My blood can save lives." Glynn et al. [49] used the expression "I enjoy helping others" in their study. They included it in the domain of *social responsibility* (prosocial, but focused on community instead of on individuals). Glynn et al. had borrowed this term from a previous study done by Piliavin and Callero [44], in which "I enjoy helping others" was found to be the most popular reason in all samples. According to these authors, this choice was an expression of "truly altruistic concerns and feelings of personal moral obligation and responsibility to the community." (p. 36) Misje et al. [35], for their part, used the expression: "I donate blood because it's important to help other people," and classified this item as an altruistic and emphatic motivation. According to Szymanski et al. [22], although the desire to help others by giving blood may emerge from the altruistic personality of donors, it is the practice itself that helps forge the latter's identity. According to Bednall and Bove's categories, and to the other researchers' interpretation, "Helping others is in my nature" could be classified as a *prosocial* (*altruistic/collectivism*) motivator (similar to "I enjoy helping others" included in their sample items), or an expression of *personal values* (*personal moral norms*).

What did our respondents have to say?

The interpretation most often shared by the apheresis donors who took part in our study clearly illustrates their generous personalities. "It's in my nature, I just like being generous. I usually prefer giving over receiving." (Male, 39 years old, Montréal, 35 donations) "I tend to like helping people."

(Female, 55 years old, Québec City, 85 donations) "I think I generally just like to help. I'm the type of person who likes doing volunteer work […] Helping is just part of my nature." (Female, 69 years old, Québec City, 386 donations)

> I am the type of person who likes to help people. It's something I gravitate towards. I am also very involved in my community. I've always been that way. Even when I was really young, I would go around collecting for food drives during Christmas time. It's just in my nature. (Female, 63 years old, Trois-Rivières, 31 donations)

In explaining why they chose this particular item, the respondents related numerous volunteering experiences they had had over their lifetime. Donating blood is therefore not the only charitable activity undertaken by these donors.

> I've always been that way. I volunteer a lot at my job. I take care of the social club. I'm actually the president. I do volunteer work all the time. Right now, I'm volunteering with young people as a scout leader. […] It's all about doing things for others […] If I didn't enjoy it, I wouldn't do it. (Male, 56 years old, Montréal, 34 donations)

Just as many respondents, however, placed more importance on the fact that they had inherited altruistic values from their families than on the fact that it was part of their personalities. It was their parents who led by example and who helped forge their identities as charitable individuals. "It's what my parents taught me to do." (Male, 52 years old, Montréal, 86 donations) "It's part of the values that my family instilled in me. It's the same for my brothers, they do other things. My younger brother is very active in his community. There's a lot of sharing […] We help each other." (Male, 33 years old, Montréal, 25 donations) "My parents are the same way. My parents were always that way. My father was always involved, both at work and with the community. My mother is the type of person who truly enjoys helping others. I think they really served as role models for me." (Female, 34 years old, Québec City, 98 donations)

In certain cases where parents' influence was cited, the respondents also added the importance of religious values in their lives. Other respondents made no connection between their family values and religious values, but directly cited the latter as a source of their generous activities. "I volunteer, I take care of people. This was suggested to me by the nuns at school. I spent 12 years [at school] with them." (Female, 69 years old, Québec City, 386 donations)

Lastly, for other respondents, giving blood or doing other charitable activities was justified by the fact that life had been good to them. It's like the principle of "paying it forward." These individuals are giving what they have received themselves [50, 51]. "I have everything I need in life, so I figure I should give whatever I can to others." (Female, 47 years old, Montréal, 76 donations)

> Life has been good to me; I make lots of money and, in return, I give lots of money to others [...]. I enjoy helping the community. I am involved in politics, I like helping people around me [...]. Donating blood today and donating plasma at Centre Plasmavie takes exactly one hour, so I can easily fit that into my [schedule]. I tend to tell myself that the least I can do is donate that amount of time. (Male, 30 years old, Trois-Rivières, 40 donations)

An analysis of the responses provided shows that, for certain respondents, "Helping others is in my nature" refers to an *altruistic* motivation that stems from personal moral or religious values (*personal values—personal moral norms*). In other cases, it seems that this affirmation is rather an expression of *indirect reciprocity* (*upstream—self*) unrelated to the fact that he or she has personally received a blood transfusion but rather connected to the fact that life has been good to them. The family influence reported by certain respondents is similar in nature: it concerns the transmission of values related to charitable actions overall rather than merely to the practice of donating blood. It is therefore part of the *social norms* (*subjective norms*) shared through the family.

"I Think There Is a Strong Need for Blood Products"

In the QBS, almost half of PPDs stated that "I think there is a strong need for blood products" (47%) was an important motivator. In comparison, only 38% of WBDs reported this item. It was the fourth most frequently selected motivator among PPDs, behind the two reasons presented above and "It's a positive thing to do and requires little effort" (52%). However, WBDs were those who most often reported this last item (62%). In the SSQI, "I think there is a strong need for blood products" is the third most frequently selected motivator among respondents (30/50). "Perceived need for donation," defined as "an awareness that blood donation is necessary for helping people" (p. 320), is a separate category in the Bednall and Bove's [7] list of motivators.

"Awareness of blood need" is an important motivator for blood donors [49, 52]. Although certain researchers have observed the importance of this motivation among blood donors, especially among apheresis donors, no in-depth analysis has been done. Bove et al. [45] pointed out, for their part, that "some donors expressed an obligation to donate, because they were aware of the medical need for plasma products, but believed that few people participate in plasmapheresis." (p. 2414) These authors note several sources of motivation for this (sense of obligation, perceived need and social norms). In reality, analyses that most often make reference to perceived needs are those that tackle the subject of barriers to blood donation: the fact that people are not informed of the real need for blood products, especially plasma-derived products, is one of the factors that explains the low number of donors among the general population [15, 16, 53, 54].

No researcher seems to have questioned how donors who are motivated to donate because they "think there is a strong need for blood" have obtained this information.

Some respondents do not really explain how they have come to think that there is a strong need for blood products. "There are people who need blood [...], you give for others who need it." (Female, 58 years old, Montréal, 200 + donations) "I know there is a need and that we should all do it for everyone, because you never know, I am healthy and giving blood today, but, one day, I might be the one who needs it, you might be the one who needs, it could be anyone. We should all give blood." (Male, 52 years old, Montréal, 86 donations) In this last example, one of the things the respondent refers to is the fact that he himself might need blood in the future, which leads us to associate this motivation to an *indirect reciprocity* (*downstream*) desire. Other respondents cited that people can become more aware of the need for blood by staying up to date on the news. "I think there is a strong need for blood because the general population is getting older and there are always lots of incidents and accidents that occur." (Male, 66 years old, Québec City, 48 donations) "There are so many cases of cancer and all sorts of other things." (Female, 63 years old, Trois-Rivières, 31 donations) "Because there are always new cases of disease, that's mostly why. I imagine that, with all of these new cases [...] we need more blood." (Male, 58 years old, Trois-Rivières, 21 donations) Hence, when it comes to the need for blood products, it appears that the responses are quite general in nature.

A certain number of respondents cited concrete examples they personally witnessed, either during their studies, as part of their professional activities (in the field of healthcare) or because a loved one had received blood transfusions. "At the retirement home where I currently work, there are dialysis patients who need blood. So, clearly, this is another reason why we have to keep giving." (Female, 69 years old, Québec City, 386 donations) When you are not personally affected, you generally don't think about it. But, when you go to [the children's hospital], it's terrible. You have to see it for yourself [...] That's why." (Female, 69 years old, Trois-Rivières, 8 donations).

> I've had this happen to close friends [...] even the daughter of a woman I know, I was her helper. When her daughter had health problems, I said "Look! We are compatible." I said "Take what you need, if you want to." When you care for someone who needs blood, you are happy they can get what they need. That's what it means to be able to contribute. (Female, 47 years old, Montréal, 76 donations)

This is the same type of argument provided by some of the respondents who claimed they give blood because it saves lives. All of the respondents who used these arguments had, in fact, chosen "My blood can save lives." These two reasons therefore seem to go hand in hand when concrete examples can be used. The argument referring to transfusions previously received by family members, however, leads us to associate this motivation to the *indirect reciprocity* (*upstream*) category.

When questioned about why they selected "I think there is a strong need for blood products," most respondents refer to the information that was personally provided to them by Héma-Québec or the information that is more widely distributed through the organization's advertising. "It's based on what you hear in the ads. That's more what it is. I really don't know anything specific about it." (Male, 38 years old, Montréal, 8 donations)

> Their campaigns really got to me. When you see that they need to advertise that much in order to attract donors, you tend to say "ok, I guess they really need people to give." [...] I tell myself that if they do that much advertising, they may not be completely out of blood, but they surely don't have enough to keep full reserves all the time. (Female, 30 years old, Québec City, 12 donations)
>
> These are things you hear a lot about in Héma-Québec's ads and at Héma-Québec's events. There is always someone there to talk about what blood donation has done for them. To talk about how it saved them.

These kinds of things make us more aware. (Female, 66 years old, Québec City, 96 donations)

It's Héma-Québec. All of the statistics they give us: "you can save 4 lives every time. 97% think about it [3% take action]." When you are an apheresis donor and forget to give, you often get a phone call, especially in the summer. They usually say: "we're low on donors, the blood reserve is low." They really seek out my help. Once, they had called me and said: "would you be willing to donate platelets, because we are in real need." That leads me to believe they are in real need. (Female, 21 years old, Québec City, 105 donations)

I used to say: "they surely have enough donations," but recently I was told "oh no, we even have to go the U.S. to get plasma-derived products, we really don't have enough." This was really surprising to me. This came straight from the staff at the blood drive and I was really surprised by it. […] It's crazy when you think that there are so many people, so many healthy people, and that there is not enough blood available. (Female, 34 years old, Québec City, 98 donations).

These references to the information provided by Héma-Québec to make donors, particularly plasma and platelet donor, aware of their need for blood products leads us to associate this motivation with the BCA's direct marketing and advertising activities (*marketing communications*).

In short, if respondents are motivated to give blood because they are aware of blood product needs, it is worth questioning what particular sources of information contributed to this awareness. When asking them to comment on the response they provided in the QBS, we realize just how strongly the BCA's marketing strategies influence this perception of need.

"It Gives Me a Sense of Pride"

In the QBS, 45% of PPDs stated that "It gives me a sense of pride" was an important motivator. In the SSQI, it is the fourth most frequently reported motivator among respondents (25/50), along with "It's a positive thing to do and requires little effort." According to Bednall and Bove's categories [7], this statement could be classified as a form of *indirect reciprocity*, related to *self-esteem*. It is similar to the sample item used by these authors in their review ("Feel good about self"). Other researchers used a different wording to express the same idea: "I expect to feel proud after donating, by doing something good" (Veldhuizen and van Dongen [24]) or "Donating blood makes me feel important" (Misje et al. [35]). Misje et al. also considered it as *self-esteem* related motivator and 24% of their respondents (active blood donors, not specifically PPDs) selected it. In the Veldhuizen and van Dongen study, WBDs and PPDs seem to be equally unmotivated by this reason for giving blood.

For his part, Healy [55] focused more on the reasons why donors felt proud about giving blood. Healy maintains that BCAs encourage donors to feel this way. Donors' pride is bolstered in part because they are reminded that few people actually give blood and that choosing to donate makes them special, perhaps even heroes (who save lives). Bove et al. [45] specifically observed this connection between pride and the feeling of being part of a special group among plasma donors: "donors expressed pride and felt that they were 'special' or 'elite' compared to whole blood donors, because this was an activity that not many people were able or willing to do." (p. 2414)

By asking our respondents to comment on why they chose "It gives me a sense of pride" among the responses available in the QBS, they were called upon to specify the source of their pride. What is it exactly that makes them feel proud?

Some respondents seemed happy simply because they were doing something good for society through this simple act: this sense of pride is fuelled by altruism. "It makes me proud because I can tell myself 'I did something good today.'" (Male, 43 years old, Montréal, 46 donations)

> It makes me proud because I am doing a good deed [...] I can be proud because what I did will help someone in the end. It's just like any other volunteer work I do. (Female, 21 years old, Québec City, 105 donations).
>
> After I've given blood, I always leave and tell myself: "I feel great. I did something wonderful." I don't know, it just gives me such joy. It makes me proud. I always feel like I've done something good for someone. Even if it's free, even if I don't know who will be [receiving the donated blood]. Yes. I definitely think it's a great thing. (Female, 31 years old, Québec City, 50 donations).

The pride motivation is associated with a quest for self-esteem (*indirect reciprocity*) in Bednall and Bove's classification [7] (*feel good about self*) who define it as "a desire to enhance attitudes of self-acceptance, self-approval, and self-respect" (p. 320). Based on the explanations provided by the respondents, one might question whether it truly is a desired effect or simply something that coincidentally occurs after the fact. This could lead us to interpret this motivation as a combination of *altruism* and *self-esteem*.

Other respondents are somewhat more specific: they are proud of accomplishing something that so few people choose to do or to ascertain that they are healthy enough to carry out a task that can be physically demanding. "I am proud that I do it because I know not everyone does." (Female, 43 years old, Québec City, 105 donations) This sense of pride is further bolstered by the specific characteristics required for an apheresis donation. "I have good blood, I am not diabetic, I have no other health problems. […] I always exceed the standards when it comes to my globules and all that, and they are never afraid to take it from me." (Male, 39 years old, Montréal, 35 donations)

> I find that, for the time it takes, it takes about three/four hours to give platelets, it's pretty long, but I always feel that this is nothing compared to how rewarding it is. Everytime I leave, I am always proud of myself. I find that it's a concrete act. To put good intentions out into the universe for everyone, that's something real and true. I feel a sense of pride every single time I do it. (Female, 28 years old, Montréal, 53 donations).

For a large number of respondents, the explanations offered revealed another interpretation: a sense of pride that stems from the recognition given by Héma-Québec or people around them. Certain respondents truly enjoy telling others about their blood donation. Giving plasma or platelets is an act that generates respect from others. "It makes me proud and my friends, parents and everyone around me is happy that I donate and that it is something dear to my heart." (Female, 22 years old, Montréal, 25 donations) "Sometimes, I'll meet someone and he'll say 'I donate platelets' and [I answer by saying]: 'me too!' I tell them the number of donations I have made and people are usually impressed because I am so young." (Male, 26 years old, Montréal, 124 donations) Donors actually have the opportunity to remind others of their actions by wearing pins or by displaying certificates indicating the number of donations they have reached.

> At first, they would give us [the certificate] in person and say "Don't file it away, display it on the wall in your office instead." It's true, people who came into my office would often say "you've given blood 100 times?" and I would answer "why, yes." People just aren't used to that. […] people don't give blood. […] When I get a certificate for reaching,

let's say, 125 or 150 donations, I display it [where everyone can see it], I am proud of it. (Female, 55 years old, Québec City, 180 donations).

It's really rewarding! I mean, when I got the picture – that's probably less important – but when I got my platinum card, I was like "wow!" The first thing I asked was "is there another one after this?" There is no other card. And, when I got their invitation, my first invitation to a Héma-Québec party, I didn't even know such a thing existed. An appreciation event, I was so happy (laughs). Who doesn't want to be appreciated? We all want it but we don't always get it. To begin, donating doesn't cost you a thing, and the recognition you get is just an added bonus. (Female, 59 years old, Montréal, 195 donations)

When I talk about this with [people at work] and say "I am close to reaching the 700 donations mark," they generally respond by saying "really?" It's really something I am proud of […]. And, when I reach my 700th donation, you can be sure that I am going to have my picture taken and put it up on Facebook. I am really proud to be able to say that I donate plasma and that I am close to reaching a goal that few [others have reached]. (Q12, Male, 49 years old, Québec City, 700 + donations).

In sum, the sense of pride that comes from giving blood can be considered a reflection of both altruistic behaviour and a search for self-esteem. In other cases, it results from the BCA's recognition activities (*incentives*) or *social norms* (*subjective norms*) produced by one's family, friends and acquaintances. The specific characteristics of plasma or platelet donation instil a sense of pride that cannot be compared to simple whole blood donation.

"I Receive Telephone Reminders from Héma-Québec"

In the QBS, almost a third (28%) of PPDs chose "I receive telephone reminders from Héma-Québec" as one of their most important motivators (7th place). In the SSQI, this statement was reported by eight respondents (9th place).

This particular reason is not often included in the list of motivators put forth by most researchers. Glynn et al. [49] for their part, referred to this as part of a specific question on the effectiveness of "following reminders" which included telephone calls. One of the respondents in our study actually referred to this reason by saying: "It's not really a motivation, I would say it's more of a trigger." (Male, 30 years old, Trois-Rivières, 40 donations) 60% of participants in Glynn et al's study [49] felt that this encouraged them to donate blood in the future. Other studies, focused on the best strategies for ensuring blood donor retention, also made reference to telephone reminders [56-58].

Why did the respondents from our study choose this reason as one of their motivators for donating blood? First off, it is worth noting that plasma and platelet donors must make appointments in order to donate blood. For some, regular telephone contact with Héma-Québec enables them to maintain this rather demanding practice given the complications of variable work schedules or health issues.

> Because I am so busy and giving blood or platelets takes up part of my week, I really have to plan it out. I can't just say "oh, I think I'll go to a blood drive, I'll be done in an hour" It's a pretty long process. I have to make sure I have a car. So, I really need to plan for it and make room in my schedule. The fact that they call me, "perfect, yes, I will make an appointment," I check my schedule and set a day and time. I really need them to remind me to do that. I am not the kind of person who can have a regular appointment every two weeks because my schedule is incredibly variable and we are often out of town. […] So, the fact that they call me really helps. (Female, 28 years old, Montréal, 53 donations).
>
> [Platelet donation] is really demanding. If I were in better [health] and more physically fit, it might be more suitable for me. All that to say that I had to put an end to my regular donation schedule […] I have not called for an appointment in several months. It is Héma-Québec that phones me, and I accept their request. (Female, 63 years old, Montréal, 19 donations).
>
> I don't necessarily call. When they call me and say: "we need you," I find the time to donate. My schedule is pretty full. So, for now, I am happy to be able to go when they call me. (Female, 51 years old, Montréal, 33 donations).

In certain cases, therefore, it seems that donors have somewhat of a passive approach to blood donation: they simply wait for the BCAs to contact them in order to make an appointment. "When they take the time to call me, I make an appointment right away." (Male, 56 years old, Montréal, 34 donations) All of these responses clearly demonstrate the influence of the BCA's *direct marketing* activities.

"I Like to Have Goals"

In the QBS, 23% of PPDs chose "I like to have goals" as a motivator for giving blood (9th place); only 13% of WBDs chose this statement. In the SSQI, more respondents chose this item (11/50) than the one presented above. Even if Bednall and Bove [7] did not include a similar statement in their sample items, it could be interpreted as an *intrinsic motivator*, considering that these authors defined an intrinsic motivator as being a "need or desire which arises from within the individual and causes action toward some *goal*." (p. 320)

As part of a study carried out among 300 plasma donors, Schneider et al. [21] asked respondents if the donation they were making on that very day was motivated by the possibility of receiving a certificate. Only 4% of respondents agreed. In the focus group study conducted by Bove et al. [45] among 103 plasma donors, it was determined that being able to donate more often is one of the key advantages of plasma donation: "plasmapheresis helped them to attain set milestone goals more quickly" (p. 2414).

When we look at the explanations previously offered by respondents during the SSQI when asked to elaborate as to why blood donation made them proud, we realize that there might be a similarity between these two types of motivation for those who pride themselves on the type of high-level goals that can be attained through apheresis donation. A cross-analysis of responses shows that few donors checked off both answers simultaneously. It is possible, however, that these particular respondents interpreted the two items as being equivalent choices. If this is the case, the proportion of donors motivated by high-level objectives is even greater than our analyses have reported.

The explanations provided by respondents in order to justify choosing "I like to have goals" as a response suggests that, for some, it is clearly a "need which arises from within the individual," which corresponds to the definition of intrinsic motivation given by Bednall et Bove [7]. "I love working with numbers and all that kind of stuff, and I think it's fun to keep track of donations and set goals for myself." (Female, 28 years old, Montréal, 53 donations) "In other areas of my life, I always set goals. That's what keeps me motivated. " (Male, 26 years old, Québec City, 124 donations).

For several donors, it is clear that this motivation becomes increasingly important over time, as they reach higher goals. "The more you do, the more you want to do." (Female, 25 years old, Montréal, 31 donations) "Well, now we are part of the more frequent donors. It's a lot of fun. And, yes, it's a bit of an ego thing. " (Male, 53 years old, Québec City, 325 donations).

> Some motivations have come over time, by the fact that it feels great to see your number of donations rise and to be able to say "I'm one of the rare few who has gotten there." […] It's wonderful. It's motivating to be able to say you are getting closer to being part of an exclusive club because of your number of donations. (Male, 43 years old, Montréal, 46 donations)

This particular motivation can also be combined with others, as is the case in this situation, where we can see two forms of indirect reciprocity (*intrinsic motivation/self-esteem*).

Certain donors recall the role played by BCA's employees who took note of their interest in setting high-level objectives and encouraged them to try apheresis donation because of this. There is also mention of the role played by the BCA's recognition activities: "Héma-Québec's reward system is really well thought out and definitely encourages this." (Male, 47 years old, Québec City, 247 donations).

> It was a nurse who worked where I used to donate. She could see that I enjoyed donating blood and that I liked reaching a high number of donations. I am A positive which I think is the universal platelet donor or something like that. So, she said: "If you want to donate more, you could become a platelet donor, have a look at this pamphlet." As soon as I found out how many more donations I could make, I was interested. So, I called right away, made my appointments and that's how it all got started. What I enjoy the most is the number of donations I can make every year. I really see it as an advantage. (Male, 24 years old, Montréal, 150 donations).

Their *intrinsic motivation* also seems to be based in the BCA's direct marketing activities. Lastly, other donors admitted that they know lots of other people who shared similar motivations and that they often seek out high-level objectives as a result of friendly group challenges. "There are three of my friends and I, and every year so far, I have managed to reach the 50 donation mark." (Q1, Male, 35 years old, Québec City, 143 donations) Each person's *intrinsic* motivations is strengthened through shared *subjective norms*.

In short, the analyses confirm that the reference to "I like to have goals" is truly an intrinsic motivation. Based on individual experiences, however, this motivation can be combined with others: *subjective norms*, the search for *self-esteem* or the influence of the BCA's *marketing communications*.

Table 6. Main motivators selected by respondents (QBS and SSQI), Bednall and Bove's motivator categories, and illustrative quotes (SSQI)

Item	QBS % of PPDs	SSQI Nb of resp.	Bednall and Bove's categories: Initial classification	Bednall and Bove's categories: SSBI Results analysis	Illustrative quote
My blood can save lives	77%	35/50	Prosocial motivation (PM) Altruism	PM/Altruism	"I do it to help others. If it can help save lives, then I think that's great."
				PM/Altruism + Perceived need	"it could be anyone. Someone who is really sick."
				IR/Self-esteem	"I would tell myself I was giving because my blood type was rare."
				MC/Direct marketing or advertising	"I remember seeing a Héma-Québec leaflet that mentioned it could help more people."
				Social norms (SN)/Descriptive norms	"My niece was explaining that platelets only live 5 days."
				IR/Upstream	"[The triggering event was] my son's operation."
Helping other people is in my nature	61%	32/50	Personal values (PV) Personal moral norms	PV/Personal moral norms + PM/Altruism and collectivism	"I am also very involved in my community. I've always been that way."
				PV/ Religiosity	"I take care of people. This was suggested to me by the nuns at school."
				IR/Upstream-self	"I have everything I need in life, so I figure I should give whatever I can to others."
				SN/Subjective norms	"It's part of the values that my family instilled in me."
I think there is a strong need for blood products	47%	30/50	Perceived need for donation (PN)	Perceived need	"There are people who need blood […], you give for others who need it."
				PN + IR/Downstream	"One day, I might be the one who needs it."
				PN + IR/Upstream	When you care for someone who needs blood, you are happy they can get what they need."
				PN + MC/ Direct marketing or advertising	"It's based on what you hear in the ads."

Item	QBS % of PPDs	SSQI Nb of resp.	Bednall and Bove's categories Initial classification	Bednall and Bove's categories SSBI Results analysis	Illustrative quote
It gives me a sense of pride	45%	25/50	Indirect reciprocity (IR) Self-esteem	IR/Self-esteem + PM/altruism	"It makes me proud because I can tell myself 'I did something good today.'"
				IR/Self-esteem	"I am proud that I do it because I know not everyone does."
				Incentives/Recognition	When I get a certificate for reaching 125 or 150 donations, I display it, I am proud of it."
				SN/Subjectives norms	"My friends, parents and everyone around me is happy that I donate."
I receive telephone reminders from Héma-Québec	28%	8/50	Marketing communication (MC) Direct marketing	MC/Direct marketing	"My schedule is incredibly variable […] So, the fact that they call me really helps."
I like to have goals (20, 50, 100, 200 donations, etc.)	23%	11/50	Indirect reciprocity (IR) Intrinsic Motivation	IR/intrinsic motivation	"In other areas of my life, I always set goals. That's what keeps me motivated."
				IR/intrinsic motivation + self-esteem	"It's a lot of fun. And, yes, it's a bit of an ego thing."
				IR/intrinsic motivation + MC/Direct marketing	"Héma-Québec's reward system is really well thought out and definitely encourages this."
				IR/intrinsic motivation + SN/Subjectives norms	"There are three of my friends and I, and every year so far, I have managed to reach the 50 donation mark."

6. Discussion

Despite the growing demand for plasma-derived therapeutic products and several countries' desire to reduce their dependency on imported products, little research has been conducted to date on the behaviour of apheresis donors. This chapter aims to better understand the motivations of regular plasma/platelet donors (PPD) in a voluntary and non-remunerated context by combining quantitative and qualitative approaches.

In the QBS, the greatest number of PPDs chose "My blood can save lives" motivation; but it was also the most frequent motivator chosen by WBDs. Previous studies [19-22, 46] have mentioned the importance of this motivation in blood donors. Although this particular wording is not the one commonly used in questionnaires for measuring prosocial altruistic motivation, it tends to be employed spontaneously by donors when answering open-ended questions and in interview surveys [19, 20, 22, 43]. Among PPDs, the second most popular motivator is the belief that "helping others is in my nature." Four other motivators also distinguish this group from WBDs: "I think there is a strong need for blood products," "It gives me a sense of pride," "I like to have goals," and "I receive telephone reminders from Héma-Québec."

The first question we can ask is why PPDs tend to relate more to these types of motivations. Certain aspects of apheresis donation help justify the choice of certain motivations over others. First off, it's a much more demanding practice because of its frequency and the time it takes to draw blood. In their comparison of WBDs and plasma donors, Veldhuizen et al. [24] suggested that "different donor profiles for whole blood and plasma donors already exist before the very first donation experience" (p. 1684). They observed that cognitive attitude was a better predictor of intention in future plasma donors than in WBDs and that "even before the first donation experience, future plasma donors were more motivated, felt more able to donate, and also expressed more positive attitudes toward donating blood" (p. 1683). In short, these results suggest that PPDs are more "driven by self" [21, 45]. It is therefore not surprising that PPDs are more frequently motivated by personal moral norms, as is suggested by the fact that they more often tend to choose the "helping others is in my nature" response.

The frequency and duration of the blood collection process means they have ongoing and prolonged contact with the collection staff members, who are an important source of information on the need for plasma-derived products or on the specific advantages of platelets. Apheresis donors are quite knowledgeable about the different uses of blood products and aware of the benefits of the blood products they have chosen to offer in order to meet the needs of the general public. PPDs tended also to be motivated more by the fact that donating blood gave them a sense of pride. Once more, this result underscores the fact that plasma/platelet donation is far more demanding than whole-blood donation. Lastly, the possibilities of making an appointment and accumulating a high number of donations more quickly are also unique characteristics of apheresis donation. This explains why the BCA's telephone reminders are more important for PPDs and why this group includes more donors who are openly motivated by the possibility of meeting high-level donation goals. In short, the characteristics that set apheresis donation and whole blood donation apart are enough to explain the results of our two studies.

An analysis of the SSQI does, however, introduce several important distinctions in the interpretation of these motivations. First off, it is important to remember that, as part of the QBS, all respondents indicated a combination of several motivations to explain why they gave blood. And, when they were invited to elaborate on the choices they made, the explanation provided for one particular motivation could easily include others (see Table 6). This multiplicity of motivators has been observed in other surveys [20, 22]; as suggested by Caillé [59], it lends itself to a combination of selfish reasons (egotism), selfless reasons (altruism, goodwill), and social obligations (social pressure), while always incorporating a number of institutional aspects (direct solicitation, or ease of access to collection centers).

The QBS results showed that almost all respondents (97%) mentioned one *prosocial motivation*. Motivations associated with *indirect reciprocity* were selected by the second highest percentage of respondents (60%) and *personal values*, the last category selected by more than 50% of respondents.

The analysis of the SSQI brought to light more complex results (see Table 6). Altruistic motivations, shared by most donors who selected the "My blood can save lives" items, are also present in the statements made by those who chose "Helping other people is in my nature." This particular combination had already been observed by Piliavin and Callero [44] and by Misje et al. [35]. The analysis of the SSQI suggests that the sense of pride mentioned by certain respondents is sometimes more of an *a posteriori* impact of an altruistic motivation than an effect consciously sought after by these donors. The combination of perceived need and desire to save lives was also observed in the SSQI; it is reminiscent of Fernandez-Montoya's [60] decision to classify the desire to save lives item in the "awareness of a concrete need" category.

Indirect reciprocity is very important for PPDs; it was associated with two of their main motivations: "it gives me a sense of pride" (self-esteem) and "I like to have goals" (intrinsic motivation). It can, however, also be found elsewhere. We suspect, for example, that donors who choose "My blood can save lives" by focusing on the sought-after characteristics of their particular blood may have been more concerned with the "*my* blood" part of the sentence. "Their" blood is therefore a significant source of self-esteem. Other forms of indirect reciprocity were also identified: 1) among those who are motivated to give blood in order to save lives or because they believe that there is a strong need for blood products, and who have found a source of inspiration among the people in their lives (upstream); 2) among those who consider that it is in their nature to help people because life has been very good to them (upstream-self) and, 3) among those who are aware of the need for blood products, and think they might need it for themselves in the future (downstream). When the personal cost is high, beliefs in personal benefits are more important for promoting actions [12, 61]. In short, donors who engage in apheresis donation seem driven more by benevolence than by altruism [62].

The QBS results do not, at first glance, shed light on the manner in which social norms influence blood donation motivations. However, the results of the SSQI suggest that they are associated with four of the six motivations analysed in this study. The people in the lives of donors, especially their families, play a significant role in making donors aware that giving blood saves lives, in transmitting values that become part of donors' personalities, in feeding donors' sense of pride and in encouraging them to meet their high-level donation goals. These findings confirm the importance of conducting more in-depth analyses of the reasons donors provided to justify why they gave blood—in reality, behind single motivations (such as altruism and personal moral values), one can often find an entire social universe that has a significant influence on the practice of donors.

Most importantly, however, the SSQI analysis results revealed the ongoing influence that BCAs had on donor practices. If, among the main motivations analysed in this study, the role of BCAs was only apparent in the importance of telephone reminders, it is now clear that the influence of BCAs can be associated to 5 of the 6 items presented (excluding personal moral norms).

These results point to the role BCAs' ongoing support plays with PPDs. In the case of many PPDs motivated by the idea that their blood donation can save lives, the analysis highlights the role of BCAs, which have long used it as a catchy promotional slogan. Staff members are also the ones who let donors know that there is a strong need for plasma, that the act of donating plasma or platelets is rare, and also that these donors may feel being part of an elite [22, 45]. Blood collections have all, in their own way, developed recognition programs for major donors, which permit PPDs to enjoy high visibility, especially when they reach specific donation targets (100, 200, 500, etc.) Special gifts may mark the most memorable moments [63]. BCAs have also developed services that phone donors to remind them when the prescribed period between two donations is almost up, and to appeal directly to certain donors for targeted types of donations; many PPDs count on these reminders. These motivators call to mind Healy's assertion that "blood can be seen not as something that individuals donate but as something that organizations collect" [55: p.71].

7. LIMITATIONS

Our data have some limitations that must be discussed. First, the two studies were conducted on samples of blood donors in Quebec, Canada, who may differ from blood donors in other countries. Moreover, we chose to restrict the QBS to donors between the ages of 18 and 55 years. The survey also tries to better understand the integration of blood donation into daily life, and especially any barriers to the practice and reasons for its discontinuation among women in their thirties and forties: this is why our sample is age-specific. The SSQI study involved an older population (up to 70 years of age). A thorough comparative analysis of the 56-70 year-old group's interviews didn't show any significant difference in their interpretation of the six motivators retained for this specific analysis, in comparison with younger respondents.

We should also point out the fact that we decided to place plasma and platelet donors together in the same group. This grouping helped increase the number of potential respondents in our studies. Other researchers have already carried out such a grouping. It was the case for Bednall and Bove [7], when they produced their meta-analysis on blood donors' motivations, and also for Ringwald and al [17], in their analysis of the reasons for non-return of apheresis donors. In Québec, donors increasingly make both plasma and platelet donations during the same appointment.

Our results were also constrained by the fact that motivations were self-reported in the QBS, which may have biased results in favour of socially desirable answers [7, 44, 45]. We should also mention the non-standard formulation of the statements chosen to represent the different motivators, which makes comparison of our results with those of other studies in the same domain somewhat difficult.

Conclusion

At a time when numerous countries are seeking to develop increased self-sufficiency in plasma-derived products, it is extremely important to acquire a better understanding of the motivations of apheresis blood donors, especially in a context of voluntary non-remunerated context. Previous studies presented a detailed analysis of motivations for a small number of donors, or an analysis of motivations for a large number of donors, but only offering a very limited answer choice list. Our study is the first to study PPDs' motivations to donate blood in a VNR context by combining a questionnaire-based survey with a full qualitative approach, using semi-structured interviews.

As we have observed, BCAs play a key role in supporting PPDs practices. In recent decades, there have been numerous studies in the field of behavioural psychology to determine the psychosocial factors that prompt individuals to develop a blood donation practice and maintain it over the long term [39]. Much less attention has been given to the influence of broader factors influencing blood donation, including the BCAs role [64]. Collection staff is certainly in the best position to identify WBDs who display those characteristics most likely to promote conversion to apheresis donation, especially those individuals who seem interested in rapidly increasing their number of blood donations and who show considerable pride in reaching specific targets. Except for Schneider's [21] and Bove et al's [45], no study has so far pointed out the importance of achieving goals for PPDs. Collection staff should also be strongly encouraged to spread information on apheresis donation, for example, by reminding people of the fact that the need is likely to grow while the country is far from self-sufficient as it is. As Kalargirou et al. [54] pointed out, this is not usually the strategy chosen by BCAs. Reminding PPDs that the organization is proud of them and that there are fewer apheresis donors than WBDs, making them truly special people, should also encourage donors. It is thus very important that recognition programs be maintained for this type of donor. Overall, these results offer points for BCAs to ponder in developing new blood donor recruiting and retention strategies.

Conflicts of Interest

The authors declare that they have no conflict of interests relevant to the publication of this paper.

Acknowledgments

This study was made possible by a grant from Héma-Québec. We acknowledge and thank Yves Grégoire (Héma-Québec) and Nathalie Vachon (INRS) for their assistance in data collection and data processing.

References

[1] Mahony, B. O., & Turner, A. (2010). The Dublin Consensus Statement on vital issues relating to the collection of blood and plasma and the manufacture of plasma products. *Vox Sanguinis, 98*, 447-450. doi:10.1111/j.1423-0410.2010.01310.x.

[2] Robert, P. (2009). Global plasma demand in 2015. *Pharmaceuticals Policy and Law, 11*, 359-367.

[3] Farrugia, A., Penrod, J., & Bult, J. M. (2010). Payment, compensation and replacement—the ethics and motivation of blood and plasma donation. *Vox Sanguinis, 99*(3), 202-211.

[4] Duboz, P., Lazaygues, C., Boëtsch, G., & Chiaroni, J. (2012). Donneurs de sang réguliers ou donneurs occasionnels: différences sociodémographiques et motivationnelles. *Transfusion Clinique et Biologique, 19*(1), 17-24. doi:10.1016/j.tracli.2011.08.001.

[5] Héma-Québec. (2015). *Annual Report 2014-2015*. Retrieved from: http://www.hema-quebec.qc.ca/userfiles/file/media/francais/hemaquebec/Rapport%20d%C3%A9mographique%202014-2015.pdf.

[6] Dubuc, A. (2014). Green Cross construira une usine de 200 millions au Québec. *La Presse+*.

[7] Bednall, T. C., & Bove, L. L. (2011). Donating Blood: A Meta-Analytic Review of Self-Reported Motivators and Deterrents. *Transfusion Medicine Reviews, 25*(4), 317-334.

[8] Anderson, L., Newell, K., & Kilcoyne, J. (1999). "Selling blood": Characteristics and motivations of student plasma donors. *Sociological Spectrum, 19*, 137-162.

[9] Julius, C. J., & Sytsme, S. R. (1993). Comparison of demographics and motivations of highly committed whole blood and platelet donors. *Journal of Clinical Apheresis, 8*, 82-88.

[10] Charbonneau, J., Cloutier, M. S., & Carrier, É. (2015). Whole-blood and apheresis donors in Quebec, Canada: Demographic differences and

motivations to donate. *Transfusion and Apheresis Science, 53*, 320-328. doi:10.1016/j.transci.2015.06.001.

[11] Godin, G., & Germain, M. (2013). Predicting first lifetime plasma donation among whole blood donors. *Transfusion, 53*(Supplement), 157S-161S. doi:10.1111/trf.12475.

[12] Godin, G., & Germain, M. (2014). How to motivate whole blood donors to become plasma donors. *Journal of Blood Transfusion, 2014*, 6 p. http://dx.doi.org/10.1155/2014/752182.

[13] Kuriyan, M., & Wells, S. (1995). Matching blood donations to type-specific product needs: a recruitment technique. *Journal of Clinical Apheresis, 10*, 23-26.

[14] Bagot, K. L., Masser, B. M., White, K. M., & Starfelt, L. C. (2015). Recruiting and retaining plasmapheresis donors: a critical belief analysis. *Transfusion and Apheresis Science, 52,* 350-357. doi:http://dx.doi.org/10.1016/j.transci.2015.03.005.

[15] Bagot, K. L., Bove, L. L., Masser, B., Bednall, T., & Buzza, M. (2013). Perceived deterrents to being a plasmapheresis donor in a voluntary, nonremunerated environment. *Transfusion, 53*, 1108-1119.

[16] Pagliariccio, A., Guermandi, G., Marinozzi, M., & Piani, M. (2003). Can better information increase hemapheresis? *Transfusion and Apheresis Science, 28*, 149-153.

[17] Ringwald, J., Lange, N., Rabe, C., Zimmermann, R., Strasser, E., Hendelmeier, M., Strobel, J., &. Eckstein, R. (2007). Why do some apheresis donors donate blood just once? *Vox Sanguinis, 93*(4), 354-362. doi:10.1111/j.1423-0410.2007.00977.x.

[18] Yuan, S., Ziman, A., Smeltzer, B., Lu, Q., & Goldfinger, D. (2010). Moderate and severe adverse events associated with apheresis donation: incidences and risk factors. *Transfusion, 50*, 478-486.

[19] Glynn, S. A., Smith, J. M., Schreiber, G. B., Kleinman, S. H., Nass, C. C., Bethel, J., Biswas, B, Thompson, R. A., &. Williams, A. E. (2001). Repeat whole-blood and plateletpheresis donors: unreported deferrable risks, reactive screening tests, and response to incentive programs. *Transfusion, 41*, 736-743.

[20] Henrion, A. (2003). *L'énigme du don de sang. Approche ethnographique d'un don entre inconnus.* (Mémoire en vue de l'obtention du grade de Licenciée en Information et Communication), Université de Liège, Liège.

[21] Schneider, T., Fontaine, O., & Huart, J. J. (2004). Ethique, motivations des donneurs d'aphérèse plasmatique. *Transfusion Clinique et Biologique, 11*(3), 146-152.

[22] Szymanski, L. S., Cushna, B., KJackson, B. C. H., & Szymanski, I. O. (1977). Motivation of plateletpheresis donors. *Transfusion, 18*(1), 64-68.

[23] Trimmel, M., Lattacher, H., & Janda, M. (2005). Voluntary whole-blood donors, and compensated platelet donors and plasma donors: Motivation to donate, altruism and aggression. *Transfusion and Apheresis Science, 33*(2), 147-155.

[24] Veldhuizen, I., & van Dongen, A. (2013). Motivational differences between whole blood and plasma donors already exist before their first donation experience. *Transfusion, 53*, 1678-1686.

[25] Weidmann, C., & Kluter, H. (2013). *Blood collection and donor motivation in Germany*. Paper presented at the International society of blood transfusion, Amsterdam.

[26] Cataldo, J. F., Cohen, E., & Morganti, J. B. (1976). Motivation of voluntary plasmapheresis donors. *Transfusion, 16*(4), 375-379.

[27] Tuleya, L. G. (2007). *Thesaurus of psychological index terms* (11 ed.). Washington DC: American Psychological Association.

[28] Kotler, P., Brown, L., Adam, S., & al., e. (2004). *Marketing* (6 ed.). French Forest NSW, Australia: Pearson Education Australia.

[29] Piliavin, J., & Charng, H.-W. (1990). Altruism: a review of recent theory and research. *Annual review of Sociology, 16*, 27-65.

[30] Collett, J. L., & Morrissey, C. A. (2007). *Science of Generosity. The Social Psychology of Generosity: The State of Current Interdisciplinary Research*, Department of Sociology, University of Notre Dame.

[31] Rapport, F. L., & Maggs, C. J. (2002). Titmuss and the gift relationship: altruism revisited. *Journal of Advanced Nursing, 40*(5), 495-503. doi:10.1046/j.1365-2648.2002.02406.x.

[32] Glynn, S. A., Kleinman, S. H., Schreiber, G. B., Zuck, T., Mc Combes, S., Bethel, J., Garratty, G., & Williams, A. E. (2002). Motivations to donate blood: demographic comparisons. *Transfusion, 42*, 216-225.

[33] Sojka, B. N., & Sojka, P. (2008). The blood donation experience: self-reported motives and obstacles for donating blood. *Vox Sanguinis, 94*(1), 56-63. doi:10.1111/j.1423-0410.2007.00990.x.

[34] Lemmens, K. P. H., Ruiter, R. A. C., Schaalma, H. P., Abraham, C., Veldhuizen, I. J. T., Dehing, C. J. G., & Bos, A. E. R. (2009). Modelling

antecedents of blood donation motivation among non-donors of varying age and education. *Br. J. Psychol., 100*(1), 71-90.

[35] Misje, A. H., Bosnes, V., Gasdal, O., & Heier, H. E. (2005). Motivation, recruitment and retention of voluntary non-remunerated blood donors: a survey-based questionnaire study. *Vox Sanguinis, 89*(4), 236-244. doi:10.1111/j.1423-0410.2005.00706.x.

[36] Amponsah-Afuwape, S. A., Myers, L. B., & Newman, S. P. (2002). Cognitive predictors of ethnic minorities' blood donation intention. *Psychology, Health & Medicine, 7*(3), 357-361.

[37] Bani, M., & Strepparava, M. G. (2011). Motivation in Italian whole blood donors and the role of commitment. *Psychol. Health Med., 16*(6), 641-649.

[38] Duboz, P., Macia, E., & Cunéo, B. (2010). Sociodemographic and attitudinal factors to blood donation in the urban population of Dakar, Senegal. *Transfusion, 50*(12), 2713-2720.

[39] Charbonneau, J. (2014). *Approches psychologiques et sociologiques du don de sang*. Retrieved from http://www.ucs.inrs.ca/sites/default/files/centre_ucs/pdf/DonSangNoteRechercheJC.pdf.

[40] Charbonneau, J., Cloutier, M. S., & Carrier, É. (2015). Motivational differences between whole blood and apheresis donors in Quebec, Canada: A questionnaire-based survey in a voluntary non-remunerated context. *Journal of Blood Transfusion, 2015*(2015). doi:10.1155/2015/568259.

[41] Moore, D. L., & Tarnai, J. (2002). Evaluating nonresponse error in mail surveys. In R. M. Groves, D. A. Dillman, J. L. Eltinge, & R. J. A. Little (Eds.), *Survey nonresponse* (pp. 197-211). New York: John Wiley & Sons.

[42] Curtin, R., Presser, S., & Singer, E. (2000). The effects of response rate changes on the index of consumer sentiment. *Public Opin Q, 64*(4), 413-428.

[43] Charbonneau, J., Cloutier, M.-S., Quéniart, A., & Tran, N. (2015). *Le don de sang: un geste social et culturel.* Québec: P.U.L. Santé et société.

[44] Piliavin, J. A., & Callero, P. L. (1991). *Giving blood: the development of an altruistic identity*. Baltimore: Johns Hopkins University Press.

[45] Bove, L. L., Bednall, T., Masser, B., & Buzza, M. (2011). Understanding the plasmapheresis donor in a voluntary, nonremunerated environment. *Transfusion, 51*, 2411-2424.

[46] Shaz, B., James, A., Demmons, D., & Schreiber, G. (2010). The African American church as a donation site: motivations and barriers. *Transfusion, 50*, 1240-1248.

[47] James, A. B., Demmons, D. G., Schreiber, G. B., Hillyer, C. D., & Shaz, B. H. (2011). Contribution of attitudinal factors to blood donation in African American church attendees. *Transfusion, 51*(1), 158-165. doi:10.1111/j.1537-2995.2010.02775.x.

[48] Beauchamp, T. L., & Childress, J. F. (2008). *Les principes de l'éthique biomédicale*. Paris: Belles Lettres.

[49] Glynn, S. A., Schreiber, G. B., Murphy, E. L., Kessler, D., Higgins, M., Wright, D. J., Mathew, S., Tu, Y., King, M., &. Smith, J. W. (2006). Factors influencing the decision to donate: racial and ethnic comparisons. *Transfusion, 46*(6), 980-990. doi:10.1111/j.1537-2995. 2006.00831.x.

[50] Godbout, J., & Caillé, A. (1992). *L'esprit du don*: La Découverte.

[51] Godbout, J. T. (2000). *Le don, la dette, l'identité: homo donator vs homo oeconomicus*. Montréal: Éditions La Découverte/Éditions du Boréal.

[52] Yuan, S., Hoffman, M., Lu, Q., Goldfinger, D., & Ziman, A. (2011). Motivating factors and deterrents for blood donation among donors at a university campus–based collection center. *Transfusion, 51*(11), 2438-2444. doi:10.1111/j.1537-2995.2011.03174.x.

[53] Gillespie, T. W., & Hillyer, C. D. (2002). Blood donors and factors impacting the blood donation decision. *Transfusion Medicine Reviews, 16*(2), 115-130.

[54] Kalargirou, A. A., Beloukas, A. I., Kosma, A. G., Nanou, C. I., Saridi, M. I., & Kriebardis, A. G. (2014). Attitudes and behaviours of Greeks concerning blood donation: recruitment and retention campaigns should be focused on need rather than altruism. *Blood Transfusion, 12*(3), 320-329. doi:10.2450/2014.0203-13.

[55] Healy, K. (2000). Embedded Altruism: Blood Collection Regimes and the European Union's Donor Population. *American Journal of Sociology, 105*(6), 1633-1657.

[56] Carter, M. C., Wilson, J., Redpath, G. S., Hayes, P., & Mitchell, C. (2011). Donor recruitment in the 21st century: Challenges and lessons learned in the first decade. *Transfusion and Apheresis Science, 45*(1), 31-43. doi:http://dx.doi.org/10.1016/j.transci.2011.06.001.

[57] Bagot, K. L., Bove, L. L., Masser, B., & White, K. M. (2014). Asking for something different from our donors: factors influencing persuasion success. *Transfusion, 54*, 848-855.

[58] Meyer, D. M., Hillman, R. S., & Slichter, J. (1984). Plateletapheresis program. I. Donor recruitment and commitment. *Transfusion, 24*, 287-291.

[59] Caillé, A. (2000). *Anthropologie du don. Le tiers paradigme*. Paris: Desclée de Brouwer.

[60] Fernández-Montoya, A., López-Berrio, A., & Luna del Castillo, J. D. (1998). How Some Attitudes, Beliefs and Motivations of Spanish Blood Donors Evolve over Time. *Vox Sanguinis, 74*(3), 140-147.

[61] Hupfer, M. E., Taylor, D. W., & Letwin, J. A. (2005). Understanding Canadian student motivations and beliefs about giving blood. *Transfusion, 45*(2), 149-161. doi:10.1111/j.1537-2995.2004.03374.x.

[62] Ferguson, E., Farrell, K., & Lawrence, C. (2008). Blood donation is an act of benevolence rather than altruism. *Health Psychology, 27*(3), 327-336.

[63] Charbonneau, J., & Quéniart, A. (2016). The influence of blood collection organizations on blood donation motivations and practices. In J. Charbonneau & A. Smith (Eds.), *Giving blood: the institutional making of altruism*. London, UK: Routledge.

[64] Charbonneau, J., & Smith, A. (2016). *Giving blood: the institutional making of altruism*. London, UK: Routledge.

[65] Kuruvatti, J., Prasad, V., Williams, R., Harrison, M. A., & Jones, R. P. (2011). Motivations for donating blood and reasons why people lapse or never donate in Leeds, England: a 2001 questionnaire-based survey. *Vox Sanguinis, 101*(4), 333-338.

[66] Shaz, B. H., & Hillyer, C. D. (2010). Minority Donation in the United States: Challenges and Needs. *Current Opinion in Hematology, 17*(6), 544-549.

[67] Zaller, N. (2004). *To donate or not to donate: An analysis of blood donors and blood donation knowledge, attitudes and practices in Northwestern China.* (Ph.D.), The Johns Hopkins University, Maryland.

[68] Harrington, M., Sweeney, M. R., Bailie, K., Morris, K., Kennedy, A., Boilson, A., O'Riordan, J., & Staines, A. (2007). What would encourage blood donation in Ireland? *Vox Sanguinis, 92*(4), 361-367. doi:10.1111/j.1423-0410.2007.00893.x.

BIOGRAPHICAL SKETCH

Johanne Charbonneau

Having received a PhD in Political Sciences from Université Laval in 1991, Johanne Charbonneau is professor at Université INRS – Centre Urbanisation Culture et Société since 1993. She is the Chairholder of the Research Chair on the Social Aspects of Blood Donation financed by Héma-Québec, the Héma-Québec Foundation and the Social Sciences and Humanities Council of Canada since 2009. She is Director of the Lien Social et Politiques Journal.

She began her career by working on such topics as the circulation of the gift within families, social and family solidarities, organ donation, as well as on immigrant communities. Her most recent works include research on blood donors' motivations, blood donation among ethnic groups, the role of volunteer work in organizing blood clinics, youth blood donors and civic commitment, and transmission of altruistic values within the family.

Her recent publications include: Charbonneau, J. et N. Tran (dir.) (2012). Les enjeux du don de sang dans le monde. Entre altruisme et solidarités, universalisme et gestion des risques, Rennes: Presses de l'ÉHESP ; Charbonneau, J. M.S. Cloutier, A. Quéniart et N. Tran (2015) Le don de sang: un révélateur des enjeux sociaux et culturels actuels, P.U.L. Santé et société; Charbonneau, J. et A. Smith (dir.) (2015) Giving Blood: The Institutional Making of Altruism, Routledge.

She has published in several journals such as Transfusion Medicine Reviews, Transfusion, Vox Sanguinis, Journal of Blood transfusion, Transfusion and Apheresis Science, Ethnicity and Health, Canadian Ethnic Studies, and Field Methods.

INDEX

A

access, 80, 135
accommodations, 104
accountability, 79
adults, 80
adverse event, 75, 76, 140
age, 10, 15, 16, 75, 108, 109, 113, 137, 142
agencies, 102, 104
aggression, 141
AIDS, 22, 23
algorithm, 14
altruism, 2, 5, 102, 104, 117, 126, 127, 133, 135, 136, 141, 143, 144
Amazon, 9, 10, 11, 12, 13, 14, 15, 16, 18, 19, 21, 24, 25, 26
American Association of Blood Banks, 27, 70
American Psychological Association, 141
ANOVA, 34, 101
Apheresis Donors, 101, 108, 134
appointments, 129, 131
arithmetic, 28
assessment, 74, 75
assets, 100
asymmetry, 41
attitudes, 18, 23, 27, 28, 41, 42, 58, 63, 78, 82, 84, 100, 126, 144
audit, 77
authorities, 3
awareness, 20, 98, 117, 123, 125, 135

B

background information, 110
ban, 91
banks, 20, 28, 70, 71
barriers, 5, 103, 109, 123, 137, 143
base, 14, 19, 76, 85
base pair, 14, 19
Belgium, 41
benefits, 5, 20, 103, 107, 134
bias, 34, 47
biological markers, 4
blame, 75
Blood Bank, 9, 10, 12, 20, 23, 27, 28, 70, 77
Blood Donation, 1, 2, 4, 101, 107, 115, 119, 144, 145
blood group, 3, 90, 91, 92, 96
blood pressure, 91, 95
blood safety, 74, 75, 76, 80, 81, 99
blood supply, 75
blood transfusion, 1, 2, 3, 6, 7, 10, 11, 12, 17, 22, 25, 26, 75, 76, 77, 80, 82, 90, 91, 92, 102, 107, 115, 119, 122, 124, 141, 145
blood transfusions, 10, 12, 25, 75, 80, 82, 102, 107, 115, 124
blood type, 90, 102, 107, 115, 118, 132
Brazil, 9, 11, 18, 20, 21, 22, 23, 24, 25

breathing, 95
brothers, 121
bureaucracy, 20

C

calculus, 42, 47, 64, 66
campaigns, 12, 18, 124, 143
cancer, 118, 119, 123
candidates, 10, 11, 12, 13, 18, 20, 26
Capability Indexes, 27, 63
category a, 104
cDNA, 13
certificate, 83, 105, 127, 130, 133
challenges, 131
chaos, 33
chemical, 32
children, 118, 124
China, 144
chronic kidney disease, 20, 23
circulation, 145
cities, 109
classification, 58, 102, 111, 126, 132, 133
cluster analysis, 74, 84, 85, 92, 96, 98
cocaine, 24
collaboration, 22, 77
collectivism, 104, 120, 132
colleges, 76
common law, 113, 114
communication, 102, 119, 133
communication strategies, 119
communities, 20, 22, 145
community, 3, 104, 107, 115, 120, 121, 122, 132
comparative analysis, 137
compatibility, 28
compensation, 3, 5, 139
competing interests, 22
complementarity, 44
complementary DNA, 13
complexity, 32
compliance, 27, 29, 77
complications, 77, 129
computer, 22
computing, 41, 48, 68
conference, 102
confidentiality, 111
conflict, 138
conflict of interest, 138
conformity, 28, 58
Congress, 70
Consensus, 7, 139
consent, 14, 80, 92, 108, 110, 111
construction, 14
contingency, 97
Control Charts, 32, 41, 42, 54, 58, 61
control condition, 43, 44
control group, 15
cooperation, 29
correlation, 63, 85, 86, 87
correlation coefficient, 86
corruption, 2
cost, 28, 29, 31, 37, 42, 128, 136
Council of Europe, 28, 35
counseling, 11, 14, 18, 20
covering, 74, 75
Croatia, 70
cross-sectional study, 10, 13, 25, 84, 85
culture, 4, 82, 100

D

danger, 117
data analysis, 71, 85, 117
data collection, 111, 139
data distribution, 34, 41, 58
data processing, 139
Data Reliability, 40
database, 14, 22, 106, 108, 109, 110, 112
defects, 42
deficiencies, 74
demographic characteristics, 110
depth, 117, 123, 136
detection, 14, 15, 21, 55
deviation, 37, 43, 50, 63, 66, 67, 68
dialysis, 124
disaster, 4
discomfort, 5, 80
discrimination, 5
diseases, 11, 21

distribution, 10, 12, 18, 21, 22, 29, 41, 59, 63, 67, 70, 71, 74, 89, 92, 98, 113
DNA, 14
doctors, 80, 119
DOI, 1, 70, 71, 72
drugs, 4, 10, 12, 15, 18, 20, 21

E

ECG, 91
economics, 6
editors, 1
education, 10, 15, 16, 18, 20, 73, 76, 77, 78, 79, 88, 112, 113, 141, 142
education/training, 77
EKG, 91
elaboration, 22
electrophoresis, 14
emergency, 119
employees, 131
encouragement, 5
energy, 107, 115
engineering, 67
England, 77, 144
environment, 17, 32, 140, 142
enzyme, 13
enzyme immunoassay, 13
epidemiology, 2
equipment, 29, 32, 33, 34
error detection, 61
ESD, 40, 71
ethical issues, 7
ethics, 2, 6, 139
ethnic groups, 145
Europe, 27, 28, 71
European Commission, 27
European Parliament, 70
European Union, 70, 143
evidence, 12, 30, 37, 76, 77, 79
exclusion, 6
exercises, 21, 77
expertise, 69
exposure, 11, 24, 25
extraction, 13

F

factual knowledge, 73
false alarms, 33, 45, 54, 57
families, 121, 136, 145
family income, 20, 21
family members, 102, 105, 124
feelings, 120
financial, 3, 5, 6, 20
financial incentives, 6
financial resources, 20
focus groups, 104
food, 121
formation, 31, 82
Foundation Center, 15
France, 1, 75
freezing, 35
friendship, 5
funding, 18

G

gel, 14
genotype, 10, 11, 12, 18, 21
genotyping, 25
Germany, 102, 141
good deed, 126
governance, 79
graph, 30
Greeks, 143
grouping, 90, 137
guidance, 75, 99
guidelines, 72, 76, 77, 78

H

hazards, 76, 99
HBV, 18
health, 3, 6, 25, 75, 76, 77, 98, 107, 115, 118, 124, 127, 129
health care, 25, 75, 76
health care system, 75, 76
health problems, 118, 124, 127
hematocrit, 40, 41, 45, 46, 50, 51, 53, 54, 58

hemodialysis, 20, 23
hemoglobin, 81
HEMOPA, 10, 12, 13, 15, 16, 19
hepatitis, 9, 11, 19, 21, 22, 23, 24, 25, 26
Hepatitis Virus C (HVC), 9, 10, 11, 12, 13, 14, 15, 16, 17, 18, 19, 20, 21, 22, 24, 25, 26
heterosexuals, 6
high school, 10, 15, 113
history, 7, 106, 109, 110, 111
HIV, 6, 11, 18, 20, 23, 24, 25
Hong Kong, 18, 23
host, 10, 11
human, 3, 4, 5, 22, 25, 26, 29, 40, 70, 71
human body, 3, 4
human immunodeficiency virus, 22, 25, 26
human resources, 29
Hungary, 73, 84
hybridization, 2
hypothesis, 20, 34, 35
hypothesis test, 35

I

identification, 20, 31
identity, 120, 142
illicit drug use, 20, 25
immunodeficiency, 23
imported products, 133
improvements, 76, 77
incidence, 79
income, 10, 15, 16, 17, 18, 20, 102
individuals, 3, 4, 5, 10, 13, 19, 25, 30, 32, 104, 117, 120, 121, 122, 137, 138
industrialized countries, 3
industry, 28, 32, 55, 69
infection, 2, 10, 11, 12, 14, 15, 16, 17, 18, 20, 21, 22, 24, 25, 26
infectious agents, 4, 12, 13, 20
injections, 91
institutions, 12, 18, 20, 74, 77, 90, 92, 96, 97
integration, 137
interpersonal relations, 104
interpersonal relationships, 104
intervention, 5, 82
intrinsic motivation, 130, 131, 133, 135
investment, 79
Ireland, 144
IRT, 73, 83, 85, 99, 100
issues, 28, 76, 77, 82, 110, 129, 139
item response theory, 74
IVIg, 102

L

laboratory tests, 14, 61
lead, 4, 50, 54, 77, 79, 127
leucocyte, 40, 41, 45, 46, 50, 51, 53, 55, 59, 60
leukemia, 118
leukocytes, 61
level of education, 18
lifetime, 109, 121, 140
light, 135, 136

M

majority, 74, 91, 112, 113
management, 2, 28, 30, 31, 32, 67, 70, 71, 92, 95, 96, 99
manufactured goods, 4
manufacturing, 28
marketing, 102, 104, 107, 116, 120, 125, 129, 131, 132, 133
materials, 5, 11, 32
measurement, 29, 33, 37, 41, 42, 47, 58, 73, 74, 83, 84, 85, 91, 95, 97, 98
media, 139
medical, 3, 5, 25, 76, 77, 123
medication, 91
medicine, 1, 2, 3, 6, 7, 77
memory, 1
meta-analysis, 103, 104, 114, 137
methodology, 27, 28, 30, 31, 34, 61, 69, 106
microorganisms, 20
Middle East, 5
minorities, 142
misunderstanding, 84

modelling, 21
models, 10, 14, 30, 34, 37, 43, 48, 52, 58, 60, 64, 66, 68, 69, 121
monthly income, 10, 15, 16, 17, 18
morbidity, 76
motivation, 11, 19, 23, 102, 104, 107, 114, 116, 117, 118, 119, 120, 122, 123, 124, 125, 126, 128, 130, 131, 132, 133, 134, 135, 139, 141, 142
multidimensional, 84, 85, 98
multiple regression, 78
multiple regression analysis, 78
multiplication, 49

N

nested PCR, 14
Netherlands, 75
Nigeria, 23
normal distribution, 29, 37, 41
Norway, 18
nucleotide sequencing, 10, 18
null, 34, 71
null hypothesis, 34
nuns, 121, 132
nurses, 73, 75, 78, 82, 83, 84, 85, 87, 88, 89, 90, 91, 92, 95, 97, 98, 99
nursing, 73, 74, 76, 78, 82, 83, 84, 86, 91, 92, 93, 95, 96, 97, 98
nursing care, 84, 91, 95

O

obstacles, 25, 141
old age, 112, 113
opportunities, 82
organ, 145
Outliers, 40, 47, 71
oxygen, 91

P

pain, 91
palliative, 118
Pará, 9, 10, 11, 12, 13, 15, 16, 18, 19, 20, 21, 22, 24, 25
parallel, 12
parents, 121, 127, 133
participants, 14, 18, 74, 80, 82, 85, 89, 92, 95, 96, 104, 112, 128
paternalism, 80
pathogens, 4, 18
PCR, 10, 14, 15, 17
performance indicator, 31
permit, 44, 55, 136
personal benefit, 136
personal values, 116, 120, 122, 135
personality, 104, 120
personality traits, 104
persuasion, 144
phlebotomy, 91
phylogenetic tree, 18, 19
physicians, 3
pilot study, 97
plasma, 3, 4, 5, 7, 35, 101, 102, 103, 104, 105, 106, 109, 112, 118, 119, 122, 123, 125, 126, 127, 128, 129, 130, 133, 134, 136, 137, 138, 139, 140, 141
plasmapheresis, 102, 103, 109, 112, 123, 130, 140, 141, 142
platelet donors, 101, 103, 104, 105, 106, 109, 129, 133, 137, 139, 141
platelets, 102, 112, 119, 125, 127, 129, 132, 134, 136
platinum, 128
PM, 132, 133
policy, 2, 7, 76
politics, 122
population, 2, 3, 14, 33, 123, 137
Portugal, 27
positive attitudes, 134
potential risk, 10, 11, 20, 21
practical knowledge, 83
preparation, 28, 70, 91
president, 121
prevalence, 10, 11, 12, 15, 18, 19, 20, 21, 22, 23, 24, 25
prevention, 76
principles, 5, 56, 71, 117

probability, 29, 35, 56, 61, 85
probe, 90, 91, 92, 95
Process Capability, 29, 63, 72
process control, 27, 28, 72
procurement, 2
professional literature, 75, 83
professionals, 77, 79, 83, 84
profit, 2
project, 69, 82
psychology, 104, 138
psychosocial factors, 138
public health, 6
public policy, 6
purines, 18

Q

quality assurance, 28, 29, 31, 32, 70
quality control, 28, 29, 30, 31, 32, 42, 54, 62, 65, 67, 70, 72
quality improvement, 69
questioning, 125
questionnaire, 10, 12, 14, 15, 21, 74, 85, 86, 101, 104, 105, 106, 107, 108, 110, 113, 138, 142, 144

R

RBC, 103
reactions, 82
reality, 123, 136
recall, 131
receptors, 20, 36
reciprocity, 102, 107, 116, 118, 120, 122, 123, 124, 125, 126, 131, 133, 135
recognition, 5, 82, 102, 105, 107, 115, 116, 127, 128, 131, 136, 138
recommendations, 31, 79
recruiting, 138
recurrence, 75
red blood cells, 103, 118
regression, 14, 15, 17, 78
regression analysis, 15
regulations, 92, 97
rejection, 33, 61
relatives, 2
reliability, 85, 87
relief, 91
reproduction, 83
requirements, 3, 27, 29, 30, 31, 36, 37, 74, 75, 84
researchers, 80, 82, 103, 104, 105, 120, 123, 125, 128, 137
reserves, 124
resolution, 75
resources, 79, 98, 100
respiration, 91
response, 7, 74, 78, 82, 87, 108, 125, 130, 134, 140, 142
retirement, 109, 124
rewards, 104, 117
risk, 1, 2, 3, 6, 10, 11, 12, 14, 15, 18, 20, 21, 25, 29, 31, 34, 35, 36, 37, 40, 42, 47, 77, 140
risk assessment, 29
risk factors, 10, 12, 14, 15, 17, 20, 22, 24, 25, 140
risk management, 1, 2
RNA, 10, 13, 14, 15, 16, 17, 20
root, 31, 32, 33, 45, 49
routes, 11
rules, 3, 42, 45, 54, 55, 56, 57, 68, 98

S

safety, 1, 2, 3, 4, 7, 10, 11, 12, 20, 21, 70, 74, 75, 76, 77, 79, 80, 82, 99, 100
sample mean, 48, 52
samplings, 28, 30, 33, 35, 36, 37, 38, 40, 41, 42, 45, 47, 48, 49, 50, 51, 52, 53, 55, 58, 59, 60, 66, 71, 85, 91, 106
SAS, 111
scaling, 84, 85, 98
school, 88, 121, 132
science, 98
scope, 30, 105
secondary education, 88
security, 75
Seekers, 9, 10, 12, 20, 21

self-esteem, 118, 125, 126, 128, 131, 133, 135
self-sufficiency, 3, 7, 102, 138
sellers, 3
semi-structured interviews, 80, 104, 105, 138
sensitivity, 55, 58
Serological Tests, 9, 10, 11, 12, 13
serology, 12, 15, 90
serum, 13
services, 6, 12, 26, 28, 70, 76, 82, 100, 136
sex, 6, 7, 17, 18
shape, 41
showing, 94, 96
Sigma Capability, 69
significance level, 41
signs, 5, 91
simple random sampling, 35, 40
simple sampling, 35
skewness, 41
skill competencies, 83
social behavior, 21, 108
social capital, 21, 24
social group, 19
social inequalities, 3
social influences, 104
social norms, 105, 119, 120, 122, 123, 128, 136
social obligations, 135
social responsibility, 120
society, 126, 141
software, 14, 18, 30, 41, 42, 57, 70
solidarity, 3, 4
solution, 40, 41, 45, 46, 50, 51, 53, 55, 59, 60, 83, 97
South Africa, 13
Spain, 78
SPC, 28, 29, 30, 31, 33, 35, 37, 42, 47, 69, 72
specialists, 31, 82
specifications, 27, 28, 29, 30, 31, 35, 42, 54, 63, 64, 66, 84
stability, 30, 37, 57, 67
staff members, 119, 134
stakeholders, 1, 30, 103
standard deviation, 32, 33, 36, 37, 42, 43, 49, 50, 52, 53, 63, 65, 66, 67, 68, 69, 85
states, 10, 11, 12, 14, 15, 20, 24, 25, 31, 33, 42, 58
statistical inference, 41
statistics, 28, 31, 41, 47, 69, 84, 85, 101, 111, 125
storage, 70
stratification, 54
stratified sampling, 34, 85
student motivation, 144
subgroups, 34, 51, 54, 58, 59, 61, 63
sub-Saharan Africa, 6
substitutes, 49
substrate, 4
subtype, 10, 18
supervision, 74
supervisor, 82
surveillance, 6
Switzerland, 1
symptoms, 82, 95
Syria, 5
system analysis, 33

T

target, 28, 106, 109
tattoos, 10, 15, 17
taxonomy, 104
team members, 110
teams, 77
technologies, 77
technology, 77
telephone, 107, 109, 115, 116, 117, 128, 129, 133, 134, 136
temperature, 90, 91, 95
terrorism, 67
testing, 11, 18, 20, 32, 33, 37, 41, 63, 66, 70, 71, 83, 85, 90, 91, 97
test-retest reliability, 87
therapy, 73, 75, 80, 82, 83, 84, 85, 86, 87, 88, 90, 92, 94, 95, 96, 97, 98, 99
tissue, 71
total product, 66
trade, 4

training, 30, 73, 77, 78, 79, 83, 84, 97
transactions, 5
transfusion, 1, 2, 3, 6, 7, 10, 11, 12, 18, 21, 22, 23, 28, 34, 70, 73, 74, 75, 76, 77, 78, 79, 80, 81, 82, 83, 84, 85, 86, 87, 88, 89, 90, 91, 92, 94, 95, 96, 97, 98, 99, 100, 145
transfusion reactions, 76, 82
transfusion safety, 7, 10, 11, 21, 76, 79, 80, 99
Transfusion-Related Knowledge, 73
transmission, 4, 10, 11, 12, 18, 20, 21, 22, 24, 25, 26, 122, 145
treatment, 5, 14, 17, 71, 80

U

UNESCO, 22
United Kingdom, 75
United States (USA), 30, 82, 102, 144
urban population, 142
urine, 91
use of illicit drugs, 10, 15, 18, 21

V

Valencia, 13
validation, 28, 37, 54, 72
variables, 15, 16, 27, 28, 29, 37, 41, 42, 62, 63, 71, 111, 112, 113, 114
Variation, 32, 33, 34, 40, 43, 45, 47, 54, 64, 67, 69, 71, 85
variations, 20, 112
vein, 77
victims, 118
viral infections, 11, 14, 20, 21, 23
virus infection, 23, 24, 25
vocabulary, 70, 71
volunteer work, 121, 126, 145
vulnerability, 20

W

Washington, 23, 30, 71, 141
waste, 33, 67
welfare, 117
well-being, 117, 118
Western countries, 2
white blood cells, 118
whole-blood donor, 101, 105, 106, 141
World Bank, 23
World Health Organization (WHO), 2, 3, 7, 100